Skills Training for Children with Behavior Problems

A PARENT AND PRACTITIONER GUIDEBOOK

REVISED EDITION

Michael L. Bloomquist

THE GUILFORD PRESS
New York   London

© 2006 The Guilford Press
A Division of Guilford Publications, Inc.
72 Spring Street, New York, NY 10012
www.guilford.com

Printed in Canada

This book is printed on acid-free paper.

Last digit is print number: 9 8 7 6 5 4 3

Library of Congress Cataloging-in-Publication Data

Bloomquist, Michael L.
  Skills training for children with behavior problems: a parent and practitioner guidebook /
Michael L. Bloomquist.—Rev. ed.
    p. cm.
  First published in 1996 with title: Skills training for children with behavior disorders.
  Includes bibliographical references and index.
  ISBN-10: 1-59385-143-X   ISBN-13: 978-1-59385-143-9 (pbk.: alk. paper)
    1. Behavior disorders in children—Treatment—Handbooks, manuals, etc.   2. Problem
children—Education—Handbooks, manuals, etc.   I. Bloomquist, Michael L.   Skills training for
children with behavior disorders.   II. Title.
  RJ506.B44B59 2006
  618.92'891—dc22

                                                                                2005022587

Illustrations by Deborah K. Reich

*To my wife, Rebecca, my sons, Andrew and Erik,
and to the memory of my father, Leonard Bloomquist*

About the Author

Michael L. Bloomquist, PhD, is an Assistant Professor in the Department of Psychiatry, University of Minnesota, Minneapolis, Minnesota. As Director of the Attention and Behavior Problems Clinic, Dr. Bloomquist provides and supervises diagnostic evaluations and family skills training services. He is a coinvestigator on several longitudinal studies examining the development of childhood aggression and the effects of community-based prevention programs, and is the author or coauthor of peer-reviewed journal articles and books pertaining to the description of and intervention with children exhibiting behavior problems.

Acknowledgments

I am indebted to many people who helped me in writing this book. In many respects, it has been a family affair. I would like to thank my wife, Rebecca Syverts, not only for her continued love and support but also for making many creative suggestions and edits. My mother, Jeanette LeVesque, did an excellent job in the word processing of the text, and I appreciate her persistence with the seemingly never-ending drafts. My teenage sons, Andrew and Erik, taught me a great deal about parenting over the years, and many of those lessons learned are incorporated herein. I am also grateful that my family put up with me as I toiled to complete this book, often at the expense of family time.

The staff at The Guilford Press have been immensely helpful. I am particularly appreciative of how Executive Editor, Kitty Moore, patiently worked with me to develop the focus for the revision of the book and shared her ideas and editing talents. I also convey my gratitude to Christine Benton for her helpful editorial assistance, and to freelance artist, Deborah Reich for the fine job she did on the illustrations.

Contents

PRACTITIONER'S GUIDE

SKILLS TRAINING FOR CHILDREN WITH BEHAVIOR PROBLEMS

Introduction

This book is a revision of *Skills Training for Children with Behavior Disorders: A Parent and Therapist Guidebook*, originally published in 1996. Similar to its predecessor, the current volume focuses on children with behavior problems but is also applicable for children with a wide array of adjustment difficulties. It is intended to help parents with a child who may be having difficulty with behavior, friendships, emotional regulation, or school performance and who may also be experiencing personal stress and family difficulties.

The book has been updated and reorganized. This edition relies less on a psychiatric framework and more on an optimistic developmental foundation. It shows how to understand challenging behaviors as developmental struggles of the child and gives ideas to get the child and family back on track by focusing on the areas requiring extra attention to bring the child back into alignment with typical development at his or her age. In addition, since the original publication, new research and practice information is available about the nature of children's behavior problems and what can be done to assist them and their families, which is incorporated in this revised text (see Suggested Readings citations).

One way to think about the kids who are the focus of this book is to view them as "struggling children" rather than looking at them as a set of symptoms that fit into a "neat" psychiatric disorder. In revising this book, I have used this concept as a major feature in looking at how children develop and run into problems. A child's behavior and adjustment problems are conceptualized as delays or struggles. The struggling child is behind same-age peers in self-control, social, emotional, and academic development, and that is

1

why the child is having problems. To help the struggling child catch up, you are provided with step-by-step instructions on how to teach your child important developmental skills that will improve behavior and overall adjustment. The parent is empowered to take charge and use skills training strategies and well-thought-out "Success Plans" to assist the child and the family. **You should view this book as a resource to guide you in teaching your child skills and learning your own skills to manage stress and improve family relationships, all of which has a positive effect on a child's development.**

This book should be read in an exploratory fashion. It is not intended to be read from cover to cover. In fact, it would be unnecessary and impossible to do everything described in the book. Rather, parents should read through Chapters 1 and 2 to find out where to begin in developing a plan of action. Parents may then elect to focus on certain skill areas first and then later on others. The subsequent chapters present Success Plans (strategies) geared toward different developmental areas that challenge a child.

The book could be used throughout the course of a child's development. When a child is 8 years old, certain Success Plans may be applicable, and when the same child is 14, other Success Plans could be used. There are charts within each chapter to aid in practicing various Success Plans throughout the book. **Parents and practitioners have permission, and are encouraged, to make copies of the charts to use.**

The following assumption about parent–child relationships runs throughout this book: Although children contribute to their own problems and account for much of the difficulty in the parent–child relationship, it is the parent who is in the best position to help the child and improve the parent–child relationship. Parenting a child is similar to choreographing a dance, with the parent taking the lead and setting the stage for how the dance unfolds. **All of the ideas and procedures described in this book involve either parents changing their behavior or leading their child to make behavior changes.** Indeed, research informs us that child-focused intervention with active parent involvement works better than child-focused intervention alone. Thus, the parent will need to work very hard to make things better in the family of a struggling child.

Similar to the previous edition, **this book has separate sections for parents and practitioners.** Chapters 1 and 2 give parents a better idea of common child struggles and parent/family difficulties and assist parents in pinpointing what areas of child/family functioning need to be focused on with a plan of action. Chapters 3–8 provide explicit instructions on how to help the child and family through a skills training approach. Enhancing a child's developmental status using skills training is difficult and may be only one piece of the puzzle that needs to be put together to help a child and family. Therefore, it may be necessary to collaborate with a professional practitioner. Chapter 10 tells parents what to look for when working with practitioners. Finally Chapter 11 informs practitioners how to work with children and parents using this book.

For many families it will be best to implement Success Plans with the help of a practitioner. It might be feasible for a parent to go it alone if the child and family problems are at the mild end of the continuum. The book should probably not be used by itself, however, to help a child or family with moderate to severe problems. In that case the expertise and experience of a practitioner will come in handy. If you are unsure how severe your child's or family's problems are, it would be wise to consult a licensed mental health professional (e.g., psychologist, psychiatrist, therapist, social worker) for an evaluation to determine if other services (e.g., therapy, medications, school-based interventions) are necessary. Chapter 10 provides information about assessment and determining a child's and family's needs.

There are several ways a parent can work with a practitioner using this book. One way involves **the practitioner helping a parent deploy Success Plans within the family.** At first glance it may seem that the Success Plans are simple and easy to do. But the author knows from many years of experience that it can be quite difficult actually to do the Success Plans. A practitioner will be able to guide a parent through common dilemmas and obstacles that come up when a family is trying to change the way it operates. The book provides an opportunity for a parent and a practitioner to be literally on "the same page" by both using this book. The combination of a parent's motivation and the professionals' expertise may ultimately be the best way to achieve results. Another way a practitioner can help is by providing additional services beyond Success Plans. Chapter 10 reviews a multitude of other interventions that might benefit a child and family. The practitioner can either provide these additional services or help the family find them. **For many families the combination of Success Plans with other mental health, educational, juvenile justice, and broader community services is the most beneficial.** This book could be used to coordinate many levels of a family's change efforts.

One caution about the methods discussed in this book needs to be mentioned. **The procedures presented have not been scientifically evaluated on the basis of parents implementing them through a "self-help" book format.** The following criteria, however, were used to ensure the methods in this book are sound. First, many scientifically tested methods that have been found effective for parents and children working with a practitioner were included. Second, the author has field-tested every method in the book in his work with parents and children over many years. This caution nonetheless is important and is discussed at the outset to make sure the parent is an informed consumer of this product.

A few words about terms used throughout the book. First, **the term "parent" is used generically and is meant to refer to any caretaker responsible for a child,** including biological parents, stepparents, foster parents, grandparents, or any adult who has assumed a primary caretaker role in a child's life. Second, the pronouns "he" or "she" and "child" or "adolescent" are used in this book. To avoid the awkward "he or she" description, the words, "he" and "she" are alternated when describing children. **All ideas and skills discussed are equally applicable to males and females.** In a similar way, the terms "child" or "children" are used throughout. In most instances, the **ideas discussed are applicable to children and teens.** Specific references to teens or adolescents are made in a few sections of the book.

It is the author's hope that parents who read and use this book will find that it helps their child and family to be more successful. Good luck!

PARENT'S GUIDE

Chapter 1

Understanding Behavior and Adjustment Problems in Children

Most parents would be concerned if they found out their child was having difficulties, such as disrupting the classroom, arguing with adults, fighting with peers, experiencing moodiness, or underachieving in school. It is understandable that parents would do all that is possible to help their child address these challenges. If you are concerned about your child, it is vital to understand and pinpoint your child's difficulties as a first step in the helping process. Once you've established the difficulty, then you can formulate a plan of action to deal with the identified areas of concern to increase the child's success. This chapter provides important basic descriptive information to increase parents' understanding of their child's behavior and adjustment difficulties.

To assist parents in understanding typical problems of children, we begin by getting to know Franklin and Jessica. Much can be learned from their stories:

FRANKLIN'S STORY

Franklin is 10 years old and sometimes "forgets" to do what he's told. With reminders, however, he typically follows directions, whether he's at home with his mom Shauna, at his dad Rick's apartment, or in his fifth-grade classroom. He was lucky enough to have his learning problems spotted during first grade, so he's pretty much kept pace with the other kids his age, thanks to special-ed classes in reading and math. At first the other kids made fun of him for having to leave his classroom and go to the "dummy's" reading group, but Franklin's parents told him to shrug it off and gave him some good one-liners to toss back at his classmates.

Even though Franklin has had troubles, he's also experienced his share of triumphs. This year he was elected student council representative for his classroom. When there's a problem to be solved, it's Franklin many kids come to because he always tells everybody to chill out and try to work out any problems they are having.

Franklin isn't going to win any awards for his athletic ability, but his Little League coach says he's the anchor of the team—the player who supports everyone else and always cheers the loudest. The day he struck out and "lost the game for the team," he felt so humiliated he called his dad and ended up talking himself out of skipping the next practice.

Franklin loves to sing in the church choir, where he sometimes has trouble sticking to the program and has been labeled the "class clown" of the group. He knows to excuse himself for a few minutes when he feels like he just can't stand still a second longer, so now he's not breaking up the rehearsals like he did before.

Franklin's fifth-grade teacher describes him at the year's first parent–teacher conference as "a joy to have in class" and says "he has good ideas." Shauna and Rick express concern that he's still only a C student. They agree to keep in close touch with the teacher. They plan to give Franklin some extra homework assignments that might boost his proficiency in specific math concepts and also to take out library books recommended for boys his age. Since Shauna and Rick are divorced, they plan on coordinating this effort across their respective homes.

"Successful" may not be the word most people would apply to a C student who isn't a great athlete and likes to fool around when he needs to pay attention. You only have to look at the bright smile on Franklin's face more often than not, listen to the phone ringing off the hook with calls from friends, and try to get a word in edgewise when you ask, "How was your day?" to know that Franklin is exactly that.

JESSICA'S STORY

Jessica doesn't follow instructions, and her parents are exasperated. It's exhausting to have to remind her constantly to do what she's supposed to do, whether it's to get ready for bed, finish her homework, clean up after herself, or even turn off the TV. Just about everything is an argument with Jessica, and it shouldn't have to be this way. She is, after all, 14.

The problem isn't limited to home either, and now her parents, Samantha and Bob, are being forced to deal with phone calls from their daughter's teachers: Jessica can't seem to pay attention without constant reminders. She disrupts the class by talking incessantly. She stares out the window or doodles instead of completing class work. Jessica's grades, the teachers warn, are taking a nosedive.

Jessica's struggles are not new. She has always been what the books label "the difficult child." Even as a baby she was fussy and irritable, and her toddler and preschool years were marked by difficulty getting along with peers. Ever since early grade school, Jessica's teachers have reported that she is frequently off-task and disruptive in the classroom. Jessica has had stretches of time where she has been doing OK. But Samantha and Bob notice that overall Jessica's problems are gradually getting worse rather than better.

Recently Samantha and Bob have tried talking to Jessica to see if they can help. Jessica only sits there looking sullen. When they pause to ask if she's listening, she snaps at them or bursts into tears and runs out. Samantha and Bob have even tried to elicit help from her much adored older brother, Danny. But she won't let even Danny into her room or her life. Jessica has clammed up, giving one-word replies to her family's tentative questions at the dinner table, and seems to be avoiding her family whenever possible. The once garrulous girl rarely volunteers her thoughts or feelings or shares stories about what's going on in her life. She seems sad and preoccupied much of the time.

Her parents comfort themselves with the idea that it's typical teenage angst and the hope that she's switched her alliance from family to friends. It's only normal, they tell each other. But they know it's not. When the phone rings in the evening, it's always for Danny. When they catch a glimpse of the kids waiting for the school bus in the morning, Jessica is always off by herself. All the tests show that Jessica has above-average intelligence, but because of the drop in her academic performance they are evaluating her to see if she might qualify for an Individual Education Plan at school.

Samantha and Bob know their daughter has a lot to offer the world. She draws beautifully and is a decent soccer player. But her sketchpads have been gathering dust in the corner of her room, and she's no longer a starter in soccer because she's "hard to coach." She's struggling in every aspect of her life, and her parents are heartbroken. They're desperate to find a way to get Jessica back on track.

In many ways Franklin and Jessica are typical of children who are experiencing problems as they grow up, although Franklin's difficulties appear to be less serious than Jessica's. This book focuses on behavior and adjustment problems in children who are similar to Franklin and Jessica. **Behavior problems** are defined here as observable behaviors that a child displays that disrupt the environment and often have a negative impact on others. These behaviors include, but are not limited to, hyperactivity, arguing with adults, sneaking, fighting, stealing, vandalizing, and breaking rules. Many children with behavior problems have other adjustment difficulties too. In this book the term "adjustment" is used generically and is not meant to imply the child is adjusting to a specific event or stressful situation. **Adjustment problems** are defined here as emotional, social, and school-related difficulties that a child experiences while growing up. These adjustment difficulties include, but are not limited to, sadness, nervousness, being teased, social withdrawal, learning tribulations, and experimenting with drugs/alcohol.

One could ask why there is mention of adjustment problems in a book about children with behavior problems. The answer is that **research and experience tells us that children with behavior problems more often than not will have other adjustment problems too.** It is therefore necessary to discuss the whole gamut of possible problems these children might have so that a comprehensive and effective intervention plan can be devised and carried out.

A child's behavior and adjustment problems can range from normal "bumps in the road" to serious troubles. A lot of children go through phases where they display problematic behaviors and adjustment difficulties relatively infrequently that nonetheless may be of concern to parents. Even "mild" behavior and adjustment problems warrant the attention of parents because the course of the problem cannot be predicted. That mild sadness can end up in a full-blown depression if the right conditions occur. A small percentage of children show signs of quite serious behavior and adjustment problems. The difficulties these children display often have a negative impact on their functioning at home and school and/or with peers.

The remainder of this chapter presents an overview of common behavior and adjustment problems in children. These behavior and adjustment problems can be thought of in terms of target characteristics and diagnoses. **Target characteristics** are important descriptions of a child's behavior. For example, "impulsivity" is a target characteristic that describes one aspect of a child's difficulties. **Diagnoses** are combinations of target characteristics to form a global category of difficulty. Impulsivity may be one target characteristic, along with other target characteristics, to form a diagnosis. If a child is diagnosed with attention-deficit/hyperactivity disorder (ADHD), for instance, he may display the target characteristics of impulsivity, hyperactivity, and inattention (defined below).

It is useful to think of a child's difficulties as both target characteristics and diagnoses. Two children with the same diagnosis may differ in the unique target characteristics that define their problems. For one child diagnosed with ADHD, all three primary target characteristics may be germane, while another child with the same diagnosis may only have problems with one or two of them. In addition, children who are having difficulty may exhibit other target characteristics above and beyond what is indicated in their primary diagnosis. One child with ADHD may also show defiance, while another child with ADHD may underachieve.

TARGET CHARACTERISTICS OF CHILDREN WITH BEHAVIOR AND ADJUSTMENT PROBLEMS

There are two important reasons parents should understand possible target characteristics that their child might be exhibiting. First, **target characteristics are "predictors"** of a child's eventual success in development. The presence of one or more of the target characteristics foretells increasing problems for the child down the road. If the child has a target characteristic, he is more likely than a child who does not have it to develop problems increasingly in the future. Second, **target characteristics are usually the focus of an intervention.** One of the primary goals of an intervention is to reduce the target characteristics. In so doing, the risk of a child having problems later on is also reduced.

Almost all children will demonstrate the target characteristics that will be described in this section to some extent. How does one make a distinction between a target characteristic that is typical versus one that can become a problem? It is the **frequency** and **magnitude** of the displayed target characteristic that distinguish between children with typical and problematic behavior. For example, it is perfectly normal for a child to disobey his parents on occasion. If a child is habitually disobedient, however, then it is much more frequent than normal and is considered a problem. It is also normal for a child to stomp his feet once in a while when angry. But if a child throws a lamp at the wall during a rage, then the magnitude is greater than usual and is indicative of a serious concern. It is a judgment call as to whether or not a child has crossed the line in terms of frequency and magnitude to label a particular target characteristic as a problem. This section will describe common target characteristics of children experiencing significant behavior and adjustment problems. As you read through this material, you may be able to pinpoint target characteristics that apply to your child.

Hyperactivity

Some children just can't sit still no matter what. They are constantly in motion and appear to be driven by a motor. These hyperactive behaviors often bother and annoy family members, teachers, and peers. Unfortunately many hyperactive children can end up rejected or ignored by their peers, reprimanded by teachers, and hard to live with at home, especially when parents are beleaguered by their own daily struggles.

Impulsivity

Kids who are impulsive don't think before acting, and often blurt out answers in class, physically shove their way in line, or even go so far as to steal something that is too tempting. These "disinhibited" children frequently have trouble dealing with strong emotions such as anger or frustration. They can get themselves into a lot of jams because of their apparent carelessness and lack of self-control.

Inattention

Children who are distracted and have a hard time focusing are said to be inattentive. It's typically not the case that they can never pay attention. Most children can watch television or stare at a video game for hours. If it is a passive activity (e.g., television) or if the child is interested (e.g., video game), then there is sufficient attention to task. If the task is difficult and requires effort (e.g., math worksheet), then inattentive children cannot muster the effort and motivation to stay focused. These inattentive children are prone to leave difficult tasks uncompleted because it is just too hard to pay attention.

Defiance

As already mentioned, it is normal for children to be defiant now and then. In fact most children ignore or disobey about one-third of the commands given them by their parents. It is a problem when a child argues or disregards adult directives more often than not. Unfortunately a high level of defiance in a child often leads to many other behavior and adjustment problems.

Aggression

Any action that harms or intimidates another is aggressive. There are many different ways that aggression comes out in children. The most obvious is **physical aggression—hurting another child or adult, such as punching, hitting, and kicking.** "Reactive" and "proactive" forms of aggression are an important distinction within physical aggression. The child who displays **reactive aggression** can be happy one minute and fist-fighting the next when an immediate situation provokes him. For example, the reactively aggressive child casually walks down the hall at school, gets bumped, and starts punching the child who ran into him. A child who uses **proactive aggression** is more calculating in his aggressive actions. This child will actively plan retaliation. In the same example as above, the proactively aggressive child who gets bumped in the hallway may plan to beat up the child who bumped him after school rather than reacting on the spot. All forms of physical aggression are more typical of boys than girls.

Children who display **relational aggression** are those who intentionally try to damage the reputation of another child. They may spread rumors or pull other kids aside to whisper gossip about a child in order to harm that child's reputation. The relationally aggressive child often tries to exclude another child from the peer group. Often, this is related to the child wanting attention or to feel superior, both of which are legitimate needs but not carried out in a way that is helpful ultimately to the child. Relational aggression is more common in girls than boys.

Aggressive children think differently than nonaggressive children. Reactively or relationally aggressive children are prone to think another child may be doing something negative to them "on purpose" and, therefore, they must be aggressive in response. The proactively aggressive child often thinks that aggressive solutions are the best way to handle an interpersonal dispute, so it is not too surprising that he would be aggressive in this situation.

Antisocial Behavior

A child shows antisocial behavior if he violates commonly accepted social standards or rules of behavior such as stealing, vandalizing, running away from home, skipping school, and/or engaging in delinquent criminal activities. This type of behavior is more typical of older children or teens. In the teen years, boys and girls are roughly equal in the occurrence of antisocial behavior.

There is a small subset of aggressive and antisocial children who are **callous and unemotional.** These children do not appear to be concerned about others' feelings and do not feel anxiety or remorse for their misdeeds. Obviously, these children have very serious problems.

Moodiness

Everyone experiences an array of moods on a daily basis. Unfortunately some children have mood disturbances characterized by either extreme depression or euphoria. Either end of the mood continuum causes problems for children. Those who are significantly depressed feel sad, discouraged, and hopeless. Those children with much higher than normal euphoric mood are often profoundly excitable, manic, or irritable. Some children cycle between moods of depression and mania.

Anxiety

Similar to moodiness, it is common for people occasionally to feel nervous or anxious. If the anxiety is extreme, though, it can incapacitate a child. The anxious child often thinks that everyday events are out of his control and is quite sure that something very bad will soon befall him. Many of the anxious child's "awfulizing" thoughts are irrational and out of proportion to what is realistically occurring or likely to occur in the future. When anxiety is severe, the anxious child may have physical symptoms without apparent medical cause, such as a racing heart, breathing difficulties, and tense muscles. This type of child may go to great lengths to avoid whatever is making him nervous. For example, a child who is anxious in social situations will feel quite distraught when in a group of children and may avoid those types of situations.

Underachievement

There are numerous reasons a child may not be keeping up at school. His lack of ability to reach his potential might be caused by neurologically based learning disabilities or might be a byproduct of simply falling increasingly behind year after year. In any event, a child who is underachieving may be delayed in reading, arithmetic, written language, and other areas of academic proficiency.

Social Maladjustment

Some children have a hard time with friendships. A subset of these children simply does not possess social skills to enable them to form and maintain friendships. Many of these children are rejected or neglected by their peers. Other socially challenged children are withdrawn and isolative. Finally, there's another group of children who have adequate social skills but associate with antisocial peers with whom they get into trouble.

One final point is made regarding these target characteristics. If a child has one of them, it is not a guarantee that he will have future problems, and indeed, these target characteristics can be diminished. The skills training strategies described later in this book, often in combination with professional interventions described in Chapter 10, can be used to reduce these target characteristics and improve a child's overall adjustment. Even if it feels like many of these target characteristics apply to your child, there are many ways to make small changes that will ultimately result in major shifts in behavior as well as self esteem and success in school.

FRANKLIN AND JESSICA

Franklin and Jessica have some of the target characteristics just described. For Franklin, the only area of difficulty is underachievement. Jessica is having problems in many areas. Accounts of her behavior suggest she is showing signs of behavior problems such as defiance, impulsivity, and inattention. In addition, Jessica also appears to have accumulated the target characteristics of moodiness and underachievement. The target characteristics displayed by Franklin and Jessica could be the focus of subsequent interventions.

PSYCHIATRIC DIAGNOSES PERTAINING TO BEHAVIOR AND ADJUSTMENT PROBLEMS

Some children display serious behavior and adjustment problems that qualify for a mental health diagnosis. The *Diagnostic and Statistical Manual of Mental Disorders (DSM-IV-TR)* a diagnostic system published by the American Psychiatric Association in 2000, is utilized to make a diagnosis in a child (see Chapter 10 for details on how a diagnosis is made). DSM-IV-TR provides information regarding all mental heath disorders and explains the symptoms a child must have in order to qualify for a diagnosis. DSM-IV-TR diagnoses typically comprise multiple target characteristics that are combined in a disorder. The child's problematic target characteristics must be beyond the normal range. For example, nearly all children feel sad now and then, but if a child feels profoundly sad it could be indicative of a major depressive disorder. For a child to be given a diagnosis, the symptoms must be observed for a specified duration. For example, with major depressive disorder, a child must have displayed the symptoms for at least 2 weeks. It is necessary that the child's problems cause "impairment" at school, at home, or within the community. In other words, to be given a diagnosis, the child's target characteristics must be interfering with his capacity to succeed in everyday life.

The main emphasis of this book is in helping parents who have children with behavior problems. In DSM-IV-TR there are three primary **disruptive behavior disorder** diagnoses associated with "acting out" behaviors in children. The specific disruptive behavior disorder diagnostic categories include attention-deficit/hyperactivity disorder, oppositional defiant disorder, and conduct disorder (see Table 1.1 for a summary).

TABLE 1.1. Disruptive Behavior Disorders According to DSM-IV-TR

Attention-deficit/hyperactivity disorder

Inattention
  Fails to give close attention to detail; careless mistakes
  Difficulty sustaining attention
  Does not seem to listen when spoken to
  Does not follow through; fails to finish
  Difficulty organizing
  Avoids, dislikes tasks requiring sustained mental effort
  Often loses things
  Easily distracted
  Forgetful

Hyperactivity
  Fidgets, squirms
  Leaves seat
  Runs about or climbs excessively
  Difficulty playing quietly
  Often "on the go"

Impulsivity
  Blurts out answers
  Difficulty waiting turn
  Interrupts or intrudes on others

Subtypes include
  Predominantly inattentive type
  Predominantly hyperactive/impulsive type
  Combined type (with inattention, hyperactivity, and impulsivity)

(continued)

TABLE 1.1. *(continued)*

Oppositional defiant disorder

Loses temper
Argues with adults
Actively defies or refuses to comply
Deliberately annoys people
Blames others
Touchy or easily annoyed
Angry or resentful
Spiteful or vindictive

Conduct disorder

Aggression to people and animals
    Bullies, threatens, or intimidates
    Initiates physical fights
    Has used a weapon
    Physically cruel to people
    Physically cruel to animals
    Has stolen while confronting victim
    Forces sexual activity

Destruction to property
    Sets fires with intent to damage
    Destroys others' property

Deceitfulness or theft
    Breaks into house, building, or car
    "Cons" others
    Steals without confrontation

Serious violations of rules
    Stays out at night beginning before age 13
    Runs away from home overnight at least twice
    Truant from school before age 13

Note. Adapted from Bloomquist and Schnell (2002). Copyright 2002 by The Guilford Press. Adapted by permission.

Attention-Deficit/Hyperactivity Disorder

This is a neurologically based mental health disorder commonly observed in children. Most children with ADHD evidence hyperactivity and impulsivity, with or without inattentiveness. A small subset of these children has only inattentive symptoms. Research shows that approximately 3–5% of children qualify for diagnosis of ADHD. The diagnosis is more common in boys than in girls.

It was previously assumed that children outgrew ADHD. Today's research convincingly demonstrates that many children with ADHD continue to have problems into their adolescent and adult years. Although children become less hyperactive as they get older, they often continue to struggle with inattentiveness and impulsivity. Children with "pure" ADHD, who do not develop other behavior or adjustment problems, often display satisfactory adjustment in their teen and adult years, but still struggle with many of the symptoms. Unfortunately many children with ADHD do develop additional behavioral and adjustment problems.

Oppositional Defiant Disorder

There is a small group of children who display defiance and argumentativeness and often refuse to comply with reasonable directives from parents and other adults. At the extreme level, these children can be diagnosed with oppositional defiant disorder (ODD). Approximately 3–5% of children have ODD, and it is more common in boys than girls.

Often there is a pattern of "coercive" interactions between a parent and a child with ODD where the parent is "negatively reinforced" and the child is "positively reinforced." Negative reinforcement occurs when something aversive is removed. The child with ODD can be so difficult that parents "give in" and allow him to get away with misbehavior. In this instance the parent is being negatively reinforced because the child's aversive behavior is stopped or avoided. Positive reinforcement is observed when something pleasurable is added. A child with ODD is positively reinforced if he "wins" power struggles because he got what he wanted (or avoided what he did not want). If this coercive interaction process is repeated enough times, the child's defiant behavior can become quite well established.

Left unchecked, ODD can lead to serious behavior problems such as Conduct Disorder (described next). Fortunately, ODD is a very treatable condition, especially if it is caught early on.

Conduct Disorder

The primary target characteristics of conduct disorder (CD) include aggression, antisocial behavior, and, to some extent, defiance and impulsivity. CD can first appear at different ages, both in childhood or adolescence, and the age of onset determines in part the ultimate outcome. Children diagnosed with CD, childhood-onset type, usually before age 10–12, often show neurologically based early aggression, along with defiance. These early aggressive problems tend to "snowball" and get worse as the child gets older. Childhood-onset CD is more common in boys than girls. Many children with early CD go on to develop significant antisocial behavior.

Adolescent-onset CD is diagnosed when a child develops symptoms after age 10–12. These children tend to be less aggressive, but still engage in significant antisocial behavior. Adolescent-onset CD is equally common among boys and girls, and its prognosis is much better. But children who develop CD in their adolescent years still have many troubles at home, at school, and/or within the community. These problems can be quite serious and continue to impact the child negatively into his adult years.

Often children and teens with CD fall in with peers with similar behavior. It appears as though "negative peer affiliations" are common in children who display CD, especially during adolescence. These teens seem to hang out together and encourage each other's antisocial behavior, which can make this behavior very tough to break.

Mood Disorders

These are emotional problems where a child experiences symptoms related to sadness and/or irritability. The child's mood difficulty causes much personal anguish. It was once thought that mood disorders in children were very rare if not nonexistent. But recent research demonstrates that children do indeed suffer from mood disorders. These children present with similar mood symptoms to adults, although they tend to be more irritable rather than down and sad as you might see in adults. This can make it tough for parents to see that their child is actually depressed, not angry or continually annoyed.

The three primary mood disorders are major depressive disorder, dysthymic disorder, and bipolar disorder. **Major depressive and dysthymic disorders** are similar, with a hallmark characteristic of child presenting with sad mood, although in some children the main mood may be irritability. These children also are likely to have physical symptoms (e.g., sleep disturbance, headaches) and experience a loss of pleasure in things they previously enjoyed. Dysthymic disorder is characterized by chronic and less intensive depressive symptoms. Approximately 2–5% of children and teens will develop major depressive or dysthymic disorders. Boys are more likely than girls to be diagnosed with major depressive or dysthymic disorders in childhood. In the teen years, however, the trend is reversed, with girls receiving the diagnoses more often than boys.

Bipolar disorder is evident when a child displays episodic or persistent irritable, sad, and/or euphoric moods. These moods are quite intense in children with bipolar disorder and dramatically interfere with their ability to function in everyday life. Not only are these children suffering from extreme mood disturbance, they are prone to unpredictable and occasionally "explosive" behavior. About 1–2% of children are diagnosed with bipolar disorder.

Regardless of the age of onset, boys tend to be diagnosed with it more than girls. When a child is diagnosed with bipolar disorder and one of the disruptive behavior disorders, the bipolar disorder is the predominant concern.

Anxiety Disorders

Anxiety disorders are emotional problems where the primary difficulty is a child feeling distressed. When suffering from an anxiety disorder, a child tends to worry, feel tense, and avoid whatever it is that makes him nervous.

The most common anxiety disorders that are seen in children with disruptive behavior disorders are generalized anxiety disorder and posttraumatic stress disorder. **Generalized anxiety disorder** is observed when a child is highly anxious in multiple situations. Approximately 4% of children suffer from generalized anxiety disorder. **Posttraumatic stress disorder** is diagnosed when a child has been exposed to significant traumatic events (e.g., child maltreatment, war, accidents) and is manifesting ongoing distress and anxiety afterwards. Approximately 1–19% of traumatized children will develop posttraumatic stress disorder. Females are more likely than males to develop an anxiety disorder.

Pervasive Developmental Disorders

Pervasive developmental disorders are seen in children who have serious social interaction problems, difficulty communicating, and often display "odd" behaviors (e.g., rocking, flipping hands, etc.). These children can be rigid in their behavior and become upset if their environment is not orderly and predictable.

The two main pervasive developmental disorder diagnoses are **autistic disorder** and **Asperger's disorder.** Both of these diagnoses describe children who have social problems and are often unable to be flexible, but the autistic child is more likely to display lower intelligence and language skills, compared to the Asperger's child. These diagnoses are rare and are more common in boys than in girls.

Learning Disorders and Mental Retardation

Several diagnostic categories are commonly given to children who are struggling in the academic arena. **Learning disorder** diagnoses apply to children who are not learning up to their potential and are significantly behind their classmates in reading, arithmetic, and/or writing. **Mental retardation** is seen when a child has limited intellectual and adaptive functioning, which, of course, also affects academic know-how. Mental retardation can range from profound to mild impairment.

Other Diagnoses Relevant to Behavior and Adjustment Problems

Several other DSM-IV-TR diagnoses also incorporate behavioral target characteristics. The diagnosis of **adjustment disorder with disturbance of conduct** can be given to children exhibiting behavior problems that are attributable to a current stressor in the child's life. For example, a child who recently became very defiant might be showing a negative adjustment to a bitter divorce between his parents. The **impulse control disorders** concern diagnoses where one behavioral target characteristic is extreme. This includes the diagnoses of **intermittent explosive disorder,** where a child exhibits episodes of highly volatile and aggressive behavior, **kleptomania,** observed when a child compulsively steals, or **pyromania,** which is given to a child who sets fires. Finally there are **V code** diagnoses that indicate a focus on a factor usually outside the child. The V code diagnosis of **parent–child relational problem** is most relevant here. It has to do with conflicts between parent and child, often stemming from ineffective parenting.

Several other DSM-IV-TR diagnoses also incorporate target characteristics related to adjustment problems within them. The diagnosis of **adjustment disorder with disturbance of emotions** can be given to children exhibiting an emotional problem that is attributed to a current stressor in the child's life. For example, a child who recently became depressed might be showing a negative adjustment to his family's recent move to another city and the stress of attending a new school. **Substance abuse/dependence** is rare in young children, but fairly common among teens. This diagnosis has to do with abuse of illicit or prescription drugs that negatively affects the child's or teen's everyday functioning. The V code diagnosis of **physical abuse of child** (or other forms of child abuse/neglect) might be applicable and relate to a child's broader adjustment.

Comorbidity

Often a child seeking mental health services has two or more "**comorbid" diagnoses,** a technical term meaning the child qualifies for more than one diagnosis. It is common that children have two or more disruptive behavior disorders. They may also have one or more of the adjustment-related diagnoses.

Similar to the point made about target characteristics, a child's diagnosis does not mean he is destined to have future problems. The skills training strategies described later in this book, often in combination with the professional interventions described in Chapter 10, can be used to improve a child's behavior and adjustment.

FRANKLIN AND JESSICA

Franklin and Jessica are both having diagnosable problems to varying degrees. Franklin's problems are milder. He clearly has reading and mathematics learning disorders but otherwise is doing well. Jessica has shown behavior difficulties from very early in her childhood and was reportedly diagnosed with ADHD and ODD. The emotional problems that her parents now observe could indicate she also suffers from major depressive disorder at this juncture.

POSSIBLE CAUSES OF CHILDREN'S BEHAVIOR AND ADJUSTMENT PROBLEMS

Although some behaviors are learned, most areas of psychological well-being are influenced by the child's **central nervous system,** which simply refers to the operations of the brain, spinal cord, and nerves throughout the body. The central nervous system comprises neurons (cells) that form neural pathways and brain structures. The **neural pathways** consist of neurons that "communicate" with each other throughout the central nervous system. The **brain structures** are clusters of neurons in different regions of the brain that regulate and control all aspects of human functioning, including those that relate to mental health. The functioning of neural pathways and different brain structures is influenced by **neurotransmitters (e.g., serotonin, norepinephrine, dopamine), hormones (e.g., cortisol), and other chemicals.**

Through a combination of genetic and environmental influences, the central nervous system of many children with psychological difficulties is subtly different than that of other children. Everybody is born with inherited genetic material that "instructs" the development of the central nervous system. In addition, environmental influences, including the family, community, and society, as well as "assaults" on the central nervous system, such as prenatal exposure to drugs, birth problems, and head injuries, exert an effect on the development of the central nervous system. It is the interaction of genetic instructions and environmental influences that ultimately determines how a child's central nervous system functions. In other words, **the mixture of genetic vulnerabilities and environmental stresses is what ultimately causes children's mental health problems.** As a result of genetic and environmental influences, the central nervous system of children with behavior and adjustment problems may be different in brain pathways, brain structures, and neurotransmitters.

A child who ends up having behavior and adjustment problems is typically confronted with many risk factors that interfere with his development. A **risk factor** is an attribute within an individual (e.g., ADHD) or a circumstance (e.g., poverty) that increases the likelihood the child will have problems. The greater the number of risk factors, the higher the likelihood that a child will have difficulties. Risk factors exist within the child, parent/family, social/peer group, and larger community/society domains (see Table 1.2). The more risk factors present, the greater the likelihood of a child developing mental health problems.

Assets and protective factors are seen in a child who develops normally. **Assets** are internal qualities (e.g., commitment to learning) and external resources (e.g., supportive relationships with adults) that are good for all children. **Protective factors** are attributes within a child (e.g., intelligence) and/or external resources (e.g., effective parenting) that shield the child from the effects of risk. In many ways protective factors are similar to assets, except assets are good for everyone regardless of risk, whereas protective factors enable a child who is confronted with risks to be successful. Assets and protective factors exist in child, parent/family, social/peer group, and community/society domains (see Table 1.2). The greater the number of assets and protective factors the greater the chance of a child displaying normal adjustment.

WHAT IS THE NEXT STEP?

Having read this chapter, you should have a good idea of the array of potential behavior and adjustment problems in children. Hopefully you have been able to identify areas of concern for your child and have a better understanding of what the problem might be.

Although it is essential to understand children's behavior and adjustment problems, it is ultimately insufficient. To be able to come up with an effective plan to help a child, it is imperative to understand a child's problems further from a psychological developmental perspective. The next chapter will provide this developmental framework. This will lay the foundation for an effective plan of action for the child and family.

TABLE 1.2. Factors That Influence Children's Behavior and Adjustment

Area of influence	Risk factors associated with problem development	Assets and protective factors associated with positive development
Child	• Early behavioral and/or emotional problems[a] • Poor social skills • Academic difficulties	• Early behavioral and emotional regulation capacity • Good social skills • Academic skills and success
Parent/family	• Parent personal problems • Parent–child attachment or bonding problems • Family lacks routines and rituals • Negative (coercive) parent–child interactions • Family problems and instability	• Close relationship with a stable adult • Supportive and authoritative parenting • Family has predictable routines and rituals • Positive parent–child interactions • Positive and stable family environment
Social/peer group	• Rejected by positive-influence children • Associations with negative-influence children	• Accepted by positive-influence children • Associations with positive-influence children
Community/society	• Poverty • Neighborhood problems • Community violence and crime • Violent media influences	• Attends effective schools • Safe and organized neighborhoods • Opportunities for positive influence: school, religious, and community activities • Nonviolent media influences

[a]Implies a possible underlying biological origin.

Chapter 2

Developing a Plan for a Struggling Child

The central thesis of this book is that a child's behavior and adjustment difficulties are best thought of as developmental struggles, and that a plan can be fashioned and put into action to get the child back on track. To lay the foundation for this approach, the psychological developmental characteristics of the "successful child" and the "struggling child" are contrasted. It is reasoned that information about the successful child can be used in a plan to assist the struggling child. The end of this chapter provides guidelines to develop a tailored plan to help your struggling child be more successful.

IMPORTANCE OF PSYCHOLOGICAL DEVELOPMENT

Child development experts have determined that the distinction between a successful and a struggling child boils down to the child's ability to move from one stage of psychological development to another throughout childhood and adolescence. **Psychological development** is the gradual accumulation of abilities and skills in self-control, social, emotional, and academic areas. The **successful child** is meeting psychological developmental challenges and is moving forward from one stage to the next. The **struggling child** is having trouble meeting normal psychological developmental expectations and is stuck or falling behind.

It is useful to think of childhood as a journey on a path toward adulthood. The child needs to take successive steps along the way, ultimately arriving at a point at which she is prepared to enter the adult world. A child who demonstrates competence at each step along the path will be successful. **Competence** has to do with a child successfully meeting the challenge of each developmental task on the path to adulthood. Each step on the path is a **developmental task** that needs to be mastered in order to proceed to the next step. A successful child is able to meet the challenges of developmental tasks, while a struggling child is not.

FRANKLIN AND JESSICA

The examples of Franklin and Jessica were used in Chapter 1 to illustrate behavioral and adjustment problems in children. Let's reconsider their problems from a psychological development perspective. In spite of some adversity in his life, Franklin is relatively competent at this time. Although he struggles with academic achievement, Franklin is happy and is functioning quite well at home, at school, and with peers. He is more likely to stay on course through his childhood journey and arrive prepared for adulthood. At this point, Jessica is not meeting developmental expectations. She is unhappy and is having difficulty at home, at school, and with peers. She may well continue to misstep along her childhood journey, arriving at adulthood immature and unprepared.

DIFFERENCES BETWEEN THE SUCCESSFUL
AND THE STRUGGLING CHILD

Throughout childhood, all children are challenged to master developmental tasks in self-control, social, emotional, and academic areas of psychological development. Parents play a crucial role in facilitating their children's psychological development by teaching and coaching them to learn psychological skills. The remainder of this section provides a description of these four areas of psychological development and the typical progression of the successful and struggling child. It also reveals how parents typically assist their child's development in these areas. For purposes of organization, the four areas of psychological development are presented separately, but in reality they overlap considerably, and a child who is successful or struggling in one domain is often successful or struggling in another. Be advised that these stages are typical and do not necessarily depict how all children develop. You will also notice that **many of the target characteristics described in Chapter 1 are descriptive of the struggling child.**

As you read below, think of your own child. **Try to determine if your child is successful or struggling in each area of psychological development.** Estimate your child's developmental age. Although your child may be chronologically one age, she may be developmentally more like a younger age. Consider whether you have been facilitating your child's development in those areas where she is developmentally younger. This will help you determine whether or not you need to focus on these areas and make them part of your plan.

Self-Control Development

The development of self-control competence involves the gradual accumulation of the capacity to follow reasonable directions and rules of adults and society as well as eventually to control internal feelings of anger, frustration, and stress. Below are the typical ages and stages for the successful and the struggling child in self-control development:

Age	Successful child	Struggling child
Infant/ toddler	• Easy-going and responsive to parent • Manageable "terrible 2's" behavior	• Irritable/fussy and/or unresponsive to parent • Tantrums and whines
Preschool	• Obeys caregiver's directions • Follows rules	• Disobeys caregiver's directions • Doesn't follow rules
Elementary school	• Usually reflective and thinks before acting • Gets upset but can calm down	• Often impulsive and acts before thinking • Gets very upset and over-reacts to stress
Adolescence	• Continues to cope with strong emotions • Aware of own behavior and its impact on others	• Frequent intense anger outbursts or anxiety • Unaware of own behavior and its impact on others

Parents can facilitate a child's self-control development by teaching her to follow directions and rules and coaching her to think of the consequences for behavior and to control strong emotions. Later chapters in this book instruct parents on how to assist the progress of a struggling child's self-control development.

Social Development

The development of social competence involves bonding with others and the gradual accumulation of social skills. Below are typical ages and stages that characterize the successful child and the struggling child in social development:

Age	Successful child	Struggling child
Infant/ toddler	• Secure attachment or bond with parent • Plays with others	• Insecure attachment or bond with parent • Plays by self
Preschool	• Mostly positive interactions with parents • Accepted by positive-influence peers	• Mostly negative interactions with parents • Rejected or neglected by positive-influence peers
Elementary school	• Good social skills (e.g., cooperative, sharing, expresses feelings) • Mostly positive interactions with peers and teachers • Affiliates with positive-influence peers • Solves most social problems effectively	• Poor social skills (e.g., uncooperative, pouting, stingy) • Mostly negative interactions or withdrawn with peers and teachers • Often affiliates with negative-influence peers • Ineffective in solving social problems
Adolescence	• Thinks of others' thoughts and feelings • Engages in positive activities with peers (e.g., sports, music, arts, recreation) • Teen "launches" from family, but maintains strong family ties • Healthy romantic relationships	• Doesn't think of others' thoughts and feelings • Often engages in negative activities with peers (e.g., drugs, truancy, promiscuity) or is withdrawn • Teen rejects family and has poor family relationships • Unhealthy romantic relationships

Parents can facilitate a child's social development by meeting her emotional and physical needs, teaching and coaching social skills, and providing opportunities to associate with positive-influence peers. Later chapters in this book instruct parents on how to assist the progress of a struggling child's social development.

Emotional Development

The development of emotional competence involves gradually learning to understand and express feelings, think rationally, and ultimately possess positive self-esteem. Below are ages and stages of the successful and the struggling child in emotional development:

Age	Successful child	Struggling child
Infant/toddler	• Mostly content and happy • Displays a wide range of basic emotions (e.g., anger, sadness, fear, happiness) • Expresses a wide range of emotions through play	• Mostly fussy and irritable • Displays negative basic emotions (e.g., anger, sadness, fear) • Expresses negative emotions through play
Preschool	• Expresses simple emotions to others • Fears are common (e.g., "bad guys")	• Unexpressive and keeps feelings inside • Fears are common (e.g., afraid of dark)
Elementary school	• Overcomes most fears • Understands and expresses complex emotions (e.g., remorse, pride) • Positive self-concept emerging • Many positive and helpful thoughts about self and others	• Fears persist • Doesn't understand or express complex emotions (e.g., guilt, optimism) • Negative self-concept emerging • Some negative and unhelpful thoughts about self and others
Adolescence	• Mostly positive and helpful thoughts about self and others • Mostly happy and satisfied	• Mostly negative and unhelpful thoughts about self and others • Mostly depressed, anxious, or angry

Parents can facilitate a child's emotional development by teaching her to express feelings and think helpful thoughts, as well as by providing opportunities for her to be successful, thereby fostering self-esteem. Later chapters in this book instruct parents on how to assist the progress of a struggling child's emotional development.

Academic Development

The development of academic competence involves exploring the world, gradually learning "self-directed academic behaviors" (e.g., staying on task, organization, completing homework), and actively pursuing educational opportunities. Below are the ages and stages of the successful child and the struggling child in academic development:

Age	Successful child	Struggling child
Infant/toddler	• Explores environment	• Apprehensive about environment
	• Is curious and inquisitive	• Avoids new situations
Preschool	• Enjoys looking at books	• Excessive television and video games
	• Good adjustment to school setting	• Poor adjustment to school setting
	• Excited about learning	• Indifferent about learning
Elementary school	• Concentrates, stays on task, gets work done	• Inattentive, off-task, doesn't complete tasks
	• Organized with school materials and tasks	• Disorganized with school materials and tasks
	• Enjoys school	• Dislikes school
Adolescence	• Consolidating special skills and interests	• No particular special skills or interests
	• Engaging in vocational or career planning and preparation	• No viable vocational or career plans

Parents can facilitate a child's academic development by encouraging exploration, promoting reading, teaching self-directed academic behaviors, and providing opportunities to learn. Later chapters in this book instruct parents on how to assist the progress of a struggling child's academic development.

Early- versus Late-Onset of Struggling Problems

When a struggling child's problems begin is also important to consider. Child development experts make a distinction between struggling children with early-onset and late-onset problems. The **early-onset struggling child** displays problems at a younger age that persist and often worsen through childhood and teen years. Jessica is an example of a child with early-onset difficulties. These children often get "stuck," and their problems grow worse in intensity and duration. Many children with early-onset behavior problems have a biologically based yet subtle brain abnormality that affects their "executive functioning." Executive functioning is the capacity to focus, stay on task, and ignore outside interference, including inner emotional states as well as the normal distractions of everyday life. If a child's executive functioning is not working well, her ability to pay attention and control emotions and behavior is often compromised. The **late-onset struggling child** displays good early adjustment with problems emerging in late childhood or teen years. An example of a late-onset struggling child is one who does well through most of the elementary school years, but gets into trouble in the teen years. For example, she may start skipping school, using marijuana, and consistently disobeying her parents. Negative peer influences and family problems are often observed in the lives of children with late-onset behavior problems. It is important to understand if your child is displaying early- or late-onset struggling difficulties so you can plan accordingly. The early-onset struggling child may require more intensive parenting and professional service efforts such as those described later in this book.

FRANKLIN AND JESSICA

Franklin and Jessica illustrate the successful and the struggling child respectively. Franklin is doing well in spite of challenges he faces in learning. He is getting along well at home and school and has many friends. Franklin's parents are undoubtedly optimistic about his future. Franklin appears to be succeeding in self-control, social, and emotional development, and although he has some learning problems, he has mastered many of the developmental tasks in the academic domain as well. Jessica, on the other hand, is having problems at home and school and is having difficulty with her peers. Jessica is struggling in all areas of psychological development. Jessica's parents are exasperated and worried about what lies ahead.

Obviously parents and the family play an important role in assisting a child's development. The next section describes parent and family attributes that enhance or impede a child's psychological development.

PARENT AND FAMILY FUNCTIONING

The parents and families of the successful and the struggling child often differ in meaningful ways. If parents and family are functioning well, it is likely that the child will too. We also know that if a parent is preoccupied with personal problems or if the family unit is having difficulties, it will undoubtedly contribute to a child's developmental struggles. Therefore, it is important to consider the parent's personal adjustment and broader family relationships too.

Parents and families can be distinguished based on how well they respond to the challenges of everyday family life. **"Coping" parents or families** function well in general and have an ability to manage daily challenges. **"Stressed" parents or families** are overwhelmed with troubles and have difficulty accomplishing daily life tasks. A goal of any intervention with a stressed parent or family is to assist them so they can cope better, which will also have a beneficial effect on the child.

Parent Functioning

Several areas of a parent's personal life have been found to distinguish between coping and stressed parents. The difference has much to do with the parent's personal functioning, status of marriage or primary intimate relationship, how well he or she deals with the challenges of being a parent, and how much support is received from others. Below are the characteristics of coping and stressed parents:

Coping parents
- Manage everyday challenges and problems
- Satisfactory marriage or intimate partner relationship
- Keep up with parenting responsibilities
- Supportive family and/or friends

Stressed parents
- Overwhelmed by everyday challenges and problems
- Marriage or intimate partner problems
- Overwhelmed by parenting responsibilities
- Limited family or friend support system

Family Functioning

Several aspects of the family have been found to distinguish between families that are coping and stressed. These include the emotional bond between the child and parent, family routines/rituals, and ongoing family-wide interactions. Below are the characteristics of coping and stressed families:

Coping family

- Close parent–child relationship
- Predictable routines and rituals
- Predominantly positive parent–child interactions
- Predominantly positive family communication and ability to resolve conflict

Stressed family

- Distant parent–child relationship
- Lack of routines and/or rituals
- Predominantly negative (coercive) parent–child interactions
- Predominantly negative family communication and inability to resolve conflict

FRANKLIN AND JESSICA

Let's go back to the examples of Franklin and Jessica to examine their family situations. Franklin was born 8 weeks prematurely, which may have affected his neurological development. Franklin's family is also poor, and his parents are divorced. But in spite of these adversities Franklin has a mostly positive family situation. Although Franklin's parents are divorced, they get along with each other and cooperate in making parenting decisions. Franklin celebrates holidays and special events at both his parents' homes. His mother has especially good parenting skills. She is supportive, consistent in discipline and rules, and provides routines for the family. Franklin's mother strives to make sure he goes to bed on time, eats good meals, and so on. Franklin is close to both of his parents.

As mentioned earlier, Jessica, who is an example of a struggling child with early-onset problems, has displayed behavioral and emotional troubles since early childhood. Her parents and family are floundering too. Jessica's parents have tried their best but admit they are ineffective in disciplining her and often give in to her angry outbursts. They both feel stressed out about parenting, and Samantha has been feeling depressed lately. They find that it is easier to let Jessica do what she wants than argue with her. The parents know that Jessica's struggles have taken a toll on their marriage. Samantha and Bob rarely have time for each other. They both work a lot of hours to make ends meet, and what precious time they do have is often spent arguing with Jessica or dealing with one of her problems from school.

Thus far, we have reviewed the differences between the successful and the struggling child and related parent and family circumstances. Parents can take an active role in helping their child to achieve developmental competence and in strengthening the family. The next section of this chapter will assist parents in pinpointing specific areas of focus and then making plans to enhance child and parent/family functioning.

RATE YOUR CHILD, SELF, AND FAMILY IN SIX AREAS OF FOCUS

Listed below are possible descriptions of your child, self, and family. Read each sentence or question and indicate how that sentence or question describes you and your child/family. Review the earlier overview of ages and stages of success in self-control, social, emotional, and academic development to be certain that you are expecting behavior for your child that is appropriate for her age. If more than one parent is reading this book, discuss each question and try to come to an agreement. Keep in mind that **there are no right or wrong answers to these questions, and they are equally applicable to boys and girls.** After completing the following ratings, you will know where to focus your efforts. Rate each question using the 3-point scale below and add up your scores in each area.

1	2	3
Rarely	Sometimes	Often

My Child's Self-Control Development

_____ 1. I give in and allow my child to get her way because she is so difficult and belligerent.

_____ 2. I have to yell, threaten, etc. to get her to do anything.

_____ 3. My child and I have power struggles.

_____ 4. I often don't know where my child is and what she is doing.

_____ 5. My child doesn't follow the family's rules.

_____ 6. There is no set time for curfew, bedtime, homework, etc. in our home.

_____ 7. My child gets upset/irritable/angry very easily.

_____ 8. My child has a hard time calming down from being frustrated or angry.

_____ 9. My child "blows up" and has angry outbursts.

_____10. My child often appears stressed out, nervous, or upset.

Total Score _____

My Child's Social Development

_____ 1. My child doesn't have good eye contact with other children.

_____ 2. My child doesn't share or cooperate with other children.

_____ 3. My child is aggressive with other children.

_____ 4. My child doesn't ask questions of other children.

_____ 5. My child doesn't ignore other children when she should.

_____ 6. My child gets into trouble with others because of not thinking ahead about consequences of behavior.

_____ 7. My child seems unaware of when she is having a social problem.

_____ 8. My child is unaware of her effect on others.

_____ 9. My child has a hard time solving social problems.

_____10. My child uses primarily aggressive solutions to solve disagreements with others.

Total Score _____

My Child's Emotional Development

_____ 1. My child doesn't seem to understand her own feelings.

_____ 2. My child tends to deny her feelings.

_____ 3. My child doesn't express feelings very well.

_____ 4. My child doesn't tell anyone about her troubles.

_____ 5. My child tends to think negative thoughts.

_____ 6. My child doesn't like herself.

_____ 7. My child tends to think things are awful.

_____ 8. My child focuses on the negative and loses sight of the positive.

_____ 9. My child tends to blame herself for too many problems.

_____10. My child puts herself down a lot (e.g., says negative things about herself).

Total Score _____

My Child's Academic Development

_____ 1. My child has difficulty reading.

_____ 2. My child dislikes reading.

_____ 3. My child watches too much TV or plays too many video or computer games.

_____ 4. My child is unable to organize school materials.

_____ 5. My child doesn't effectively budget her time.

_____ 6. My child often doesn't know what homework she is supposed to do.

_____ 7. My child is usually off task and doesn't get much work done at school.

_____ 8. My child is usually off task and doesn't get much homework done at home.

_____ 9. My child has poor study skills and habits.

_____10. My child doesn't have a routine time or designated place for homework.

Total Score _____

My Personal Well-Being as a Parent

_____ 1. I feel overwhelmed with responsibilities.

_____ 2. I feel depressed and unhappy.

_____ 3. I use alcohol and/or drugs too often.

_____ 4. I find my child to be too difficult to discipline.

_____ 5. I feel like I have no support and I'm all alone.

_____ 6. I often have a thought like, "My child is behaving like a brat."

_____ 7. I often have a thought like, "My child does it on purpose."

_____ 8. I often have a thought like, "My child's future is bleak, and she is going to have problems as an adult."

_____ 9. I often have a thought like, "I give up; there is nothing more I can do for my child."

_____10. I often have a thought like, "I have no control over my child. I've tried everything; nothing seems to work."

Total Score _____

My Family's Relationships

_____ 1. I don't pay much attention to my child's good behavior.

_____ 2. I have more negative interactions than positive interactions with my child.

_____ 3. We don't have daily routines and/or a schedule in our home.

_____ 4. I'm not involved in my child's activities. (e.g., school, athletics, scouts, etc.).

_____ 5. My child and I are not very close to each other.

_____ 6. We express ourselves in "unhelpful" ways in our family (e.g., put downs, blaming, interrupting).

_____ 7. We are not good at listening to each other. (e.g., make poor eye contact, daydream, think about what one is going to say without listening to the other person).

_____ 8. We have difficulty recognizing and defining our family problems.

_____ 9. We usually don't recognize when anger and conflict are becoming destructive.

_____10. Anger and conflict get out of control in our family.

Total Score _____

Review your answers to the above questions carefully. Add up the score within each of the six areas of focus and write in the total score. **Those areas of focus with higher scores may indicate problem areas for your child, self, and/or family, while those questions that were rated as a 3 may indicate specific problems.**

DECIDING ON AN AREA OF FOCUS

In the space below rank the six areas of focus, putting the area with the highest score on top, going down to the second highest score, and so on until you have ranked all six areas of focus.

1. _____

2. _____

3. _____

4. _____

5. _____

6. _____

By ranking the six areas of focus by their scores, you are making use of a scientific method. Now examine the list again and use your gut reaction to rank the areas according to the ones you think are the most important to focus on. Keep in mind that it is usually less effective to focus on the child if the parent or family is having problems. **It may be wise to focus on parent and family areas before or at the same time as the child.**

HOW TO USE THIS BOOK

Now that you have determined an area of focus, you can plan to assist your child and family. This can be accomplished by teaching your child developmental skills, taking care of your parent and family stress, keeping it going, and seeking professional help if needed. Different chapters in this book offer step-by-step instructions for implementing *Success Plans* to help your child, self, and family. Below is a brief overview of the Success Plans that are described in greater detail throughout the book.

Teaching Your Child Developmental Skills

Children learn the tasks for successful development gradually as they get older. If you have determined that your child is delayed in a certain area of development, she needs to be taught those skills. If your child is struggling, you can teach her skills to catch up and become more successful in self-control, social, emotional, and academic areas of focus. In turn, your child should display a decline in behavioral and adjustment problems. The Child Success Plans listed below (see Figure 2.1) need to be selected to match the developmental age of the child. In other words, **it is best to plan according to how the child functions developmentally** (see Chapter 1) instead of by the child's actual chronological age. The corresponding chapters for each Child Success Plan provide further guidance to parents.

Taking Care of Parent and Family Stress

It is important to remember that it will be difficult to teach a child important developmental skills if the parent or family is too stressed out. If you think you or your family are having difficulty, it is important to address those problems before or at the same time the child is taught new skills. You can employ Parent and Family Success Plans listed below (see Figure 2.2) to improve par-

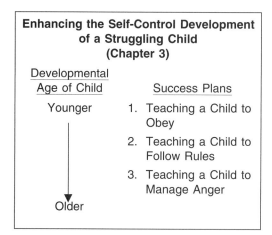

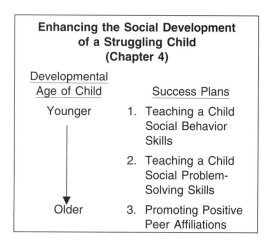

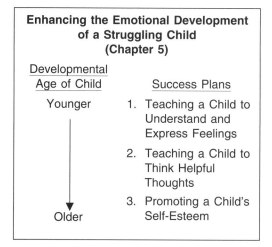

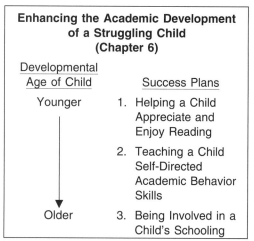

FIGURE 2.1. Child Success Plans.

ent and family functioning. The corresponding chapters for each Parent and Family Success Plan provide further guidance to parents.

Keeping It Going

Keep in mind that implementing any Success Plan described in this book will require a lot of effort on your part. The old saying **"no pain, no gain"** applies here. You need to put in the effort if you really want to make changes for your child, self, and/or family. It is helpful to think of long-term benefits rather than short-term gains. If you put in the effort now, it could potentially pay off

Improving Parent Well-Being (Chapter 7)		Improving Family Relationships (Chapter 8)	
Developmental Age of Child	Success Plans	Developmental Age of Child	Success Plans
All Ages	1. Improving Parent Stress Management Skills	All Ages	1. Improving the Parent–Child Bond
	2. Staying Calm with a Stressful Child		2. Improving Family Interactions
	3. Changing Unhelpful Parent Thoughts		3. Developing Family Routines and Rituals

FIGURE 2.2. Parent and Family Success Plans.

in the long run. It is also necessary to keep in mind that, sometimes, when trying new plans, old problems get worse before they get better. You will see positive results, however, if you stay with it long enough to make it work. Unfortunately it is human nature to start up new endeavors and let them fall by the wayside. The Success Plans described in Chapters 3 through 8 require **consistent and persistent effort** to make them work. Chapter 9 offers common-sense suggestions to keep it going over the long haul.

Seeking Professional Help

Sometimes a child's, parent's, or family's problems are of a serious nature. Although the Success Plans may help, they may not be enough. Fortunately families can access professional help within mental health agencies, schools, juvenile courts, and communities to assist when challenges are significant. Chapter 10 provides information about what to look for when seeking effective professional services.

REASON FOR HOPE

There are no guarantees with children. It is safe to assume, however, that if you faithfully try to apply the Success Plans outlined in the book and seek out other professional services if needed, then the odds of overcoming a child's behavioral and adjustment problems are greatly enhanced. In other words, there is reason for hope.

To understand why there is reason for hope, it may be helpful to review the end of Chapter 1, which was about possible causes of children's behavior and adjustment problems. Table 1.2 in Chapter 1 summarized the risk factors observed in children with problems and the assets and protective factors often seen in children who are better adjusted. By employing the ideas in this book, you will in effect be reducing risk factors and increasing assets and protective factors, which should result in better behavior and adjustment in your child.

Chapter 3

Enhancing a Child's Self-Control Development

Self-control problems in a struggling child often take the form of disobedience of reasonable adult directives, violations of commonly accepted rules, or trouble dealing with anger. These are potentially serious problems because children who routinely demonstrate these behaviors are often rejected by positive peers, have school adjustment problems, and may eventually become involved in delinquent behavior or develop emotional problems. To be successful, a child must first be "externally controlled" by adults (follow directions and rules) and then gradually mature to being "internally controlled" (handling strong emotions).

It should be pointed out that the development of self-control also depends on possessing good social and emotional skills. A child who learns how to get along with others and express feelings will have better self-control. Therefore, to enhance your child's self-control development, you may also want to work to improve your child's social and emotional skills as described in Chapters 4 and 5.

This chapter provides three Child Self-Control Success Plans for a parent to facilitate self-control development in a struggling child:

Child Self-Control Success Plan 1: Teaching a Child to Obey—gives ideas to increase the rates of a child's obedience with reasonable parental directives (see pages 44–49).

Child Self-Control Success Plan 2: Teaching a Child to Follow Rules—

provides methods to define rules and improve the child's inclination for following them (see pages 50–53).

Child Self-Control Success Plan 3: Teaching a Child to Manage Anger— focuses on assisting a child to manage strong feelings of frustration and anger (see pages 53–58).

Each of these Child Self-Control Success Plans will be useful for a child at different ages. Child Self-Control Success Plans 1 and 2 are helpful for a younger child or an older child/teen who hasn't yet learned to obey and follow rules. Child Self-Control Success Plan 3 is best suited for an older child/ teen who is relatively good at obeying and following rules and who possesses some advanced thinking skills necessary to learn the relatively complex anger management skills. If you are uncertain of your child's level of self-control development, consult Chapter 2 for more details.

A parent might want to work with a child on all self-control skills in turn. For example, it may be useful to focus on teaching a child to obey for several weeks or months, to follow rules for several weeks or months, and then, if the child is old enough, anger management skills.

CHILD SELF-CONTROL SUCCESS PLAN 1: TEACHING A CHILD TO OBEY

CAN'T YOU DO WHAT I TELL YOU?

Dan is a single parent who is trying to raise his 10-year-old daughter, Shelby. He complains that he can't get Shelby to do anything. He has to tell her over and over to do simple things that "kids her age should be able to do." Is it too much, Dan wonders, to expect a 10-year-old girl to make her bed each day and complete her homework? He finds himself yelling at Shelby and saying things to her that he often later regrets. Shelby routinely is argumentative, talks back, or tries to blame him for being "unfair."

Removal of Privileges for Disobedience

On a typical day a parent might state literally hundreds of commands to his or her child. These directives can be as benign as "pass the milk" or as important as "go to bed" or "do your homework." Most children will ignore or even defy their parent's instructions occasionally. If a child is habitually disobedient, however, then it is a problem that needs to be addressed. Most children will comply with parents' commands about two-thirds of the time, so it is "normal" for children to be noncompliant about one-third of the time. The procedures described in this section are useful to improve any child's level of obedience, but can be especially helpful for children with higher than average rates of noncompliance.

To begin, let's examine the sequence of events that typically occurs in a situation where a child should obey. Usually a parent tells a child to do something. Then, in response to that directive, the child does or does not do what he is told. In some households, if the child is disobedient, the parent may yell and threaten until the child is compliant or just forget about it and withdraw the original command because it is not worth the hassle and stress. Unfortunately these parent and child behaviors can become a pattern. To break the habit, it's up to the parent to change his or her behavior first. The parent must lead the child toward greater obedience.

Next let's make sure you completely understand what disobedience is so that when you see it you know it is time to take action. Disobedience is broadly defined as a child resisting or refusing to follow a parental directive. But there are three common variations on the disobedience theme in children:

- **Overt noncompliance**—where the child refuses to perform the task physically (e.g., parent instructs child to turn off TV, and child says "No").
- **Bargaining**—the child verbally tries to strike up a deal with the parent, but is not complying with the command (e.g., "How about I do it after this TV show?")
- **Resistance**—the child complains and half-heartedly complies with the request (e.g., parent directs child to clean up his room; he complains and whines, goes in the room, picks up a toy here and there, but never really accomplishes the task).

Whenever you observe these three types of disobedience you should try to use the steps articulated below.

Step 1: Give Effective Commands

As stated earlier, disobedience occurs when a child is told to do something and does not do it. **It may be helpful to think about whether the way you tell**

your child to do something may be contributing to the problem. Read the list of commands below and consider which of them are typical of you:

- **Vague command:** Telling a child in vague terms what he is expected to do (e.g., "Shape up" or "Knock it off").
- **Question command:** Asking a question in an attempt to gain a child's compliance (e.g., "Would you please pick up your toys?").
- **Rationale command:** Explaining to a child why he needs to comply (e.g., "You need to get dressed now, because if you don't we will be late for our appointment").
- **Multiple commands:** Telling a child to do too many things at once (e.g., "Pick up your toys, make your bed, wash your hands, and then come to dinner").
- **Frequent commands:** Repeating the same command over and over to a child.
- **Specific, one-step command:** Stating a specific, one-step command in 10 words or less (e.g., "Turn off the TV now").

You may have already guessed that **vague, question, rationale, multiple, and frequent commands are not very effective with disobedient children.** This is not to say that a parent should never ask a question or present a rationale, but it is unwise to do so at moments where the goal is to have the child obey. Try to avoid using those ineffective commands in situations where you expect your child to comply. A vague command does not tell a child specifically what he is expected to do. A question command doesn't work because a child is given the option to comply or not as stated in the question. A rationale command is problematic because a child may choose to dispute the rationale rather than comply with the command (e.g., "We have plenty of time. We won't be late."). Multiple commands are difficult for a child because he may become overwhelmed and/or confused by the many steps of the command. The frequent command is ineffective because a child learns that the parent does not necessarily mean it when the command is stated the first time.

In contrast, **the specific, one-step command stated in 10 words or less helps a child be more compliant** because it tells a child exactly what is expected of him. For the specific command to be most effective, it should be stated only once. It also helps to ask your child for eye contact and to raise your voice *slightly* while stating it. Strive to give specific, one-step commands in this manner when you want your child to comply. **Be sure to praise your child if he complies with your command.**

Step 2: Use Effective Warnings

If your child does not comply with an effective command, it is necessary to give him a warning. **The best way to state a warning is in the form of an "if . . . then" statement.** For example, if a child refuses your command to "turn off the TV now," you should say, "**if** you don't turn off the TV now, **then** you will (have a privilege removed)." "If . . . then" statements clearly tell the child what will happen if he doesn't comply. It's also very important to **state the warning only once.** Similar to the command, when giving a warning, it helps to look into your child's eyes and raise your voice *slightly* while stating it. If you are consistent in giving only one warning, eventually your child will learn to comply with your warning and it will be unnecessary to go to Step 3 below (removal of a privilege). It may be helpful to state the warning and count out loud to 3 before following through with Step 3. **Be sure to praise your child if he complies with your warning.**

Step 3: Take Away a Privilege If Child Does Not Comply with Warning

This step involves following through with the warning stated in Step 2 above. You take away a privilege from your child because he did not obey your command or heed your warning. Removing a privilege will inform and teach your child that you are serious about him needing to obey. Privileges that are taken away can vary according to the circumstance and child's age.

It is recommended to use a time-out chair if you have time and if your child is at the preschool or elementary school age (roughly 3–10 years old). The time-out chair is a variation on removal of privileges because when in a time-out chair, the child loses the privilege of interaction with his parents and access to toys, games, TV, and so forth. If the child does not comply with the warning, then immediately put the child in the designated time-out chair. The time-out chair should be located in a place where there is nothing to distract or entertain the child (e.g., corner of a room, a hallway). The child is required to sit in the chair for a specified length of time. It may be helpful to set a timer for 2 to 5 minutes (the parent should judge what an adequate time length is and utilize the same time length for every time-out). It is okay if the child protests a little, as long as he sits in the chair. **If the child leaves the chair or acts in a severely disruptive manner, the parent should warn him that the timer will be set back until he sits in the chair quietly.** If the child continues to act up in the time-out chair, restart the timer. If the child's time-out behavior does not improve after several tries of resetting the timer, the parent may have to use a consequence such as taking away a future privilege. For example, if the child doesn't sit in the chair, he will not be allowed to watch TV until he does. If the child is then able to sit quietly, set the timer again for the designated time period. Once the child has satisfied the requirements for the time-out chair, then he can be released, along with the parent restating the original command.

If you do not have time (e.g., you are rushing to get to work) and/or if your child is older or a teen it is a good idea to take away "extra privileges." These extra privileges could include, but are not limited to, TV, computer, stereo, going outside, games, toys, driving the car, and so on. These privileges are what the child or teen enjoys but does not necessarily need. The child or teen is told that **if** he doesn't obey the command, **then** he will lose an extra privilege for a specified period of time according to two options:

> **Option 1:** The child/teen is told that the privilege is lost until he is compliant with the original command (e.g., no TV until homework is done).
> **Option 2:** The child/teen is told the privilege is lost for a specified period of time (e.g., no TV for 24 hours).

Once the child or teen has satisfied the requirements for the loss of extra privilege, then he can retain the privilege once again, along with the parent restating the original command.

Step 4: Calm Down and Stay Cool

A disobedient child is very challenging, and his parent often gets angry, yells, and sometimes resorts to physical punishment. It is extremely important to **calm down and stay cool** to avoid power struggles. Try to maintain a matter-of-fact, composed demeanor. Some parents imagine themselves as a robot that goes through the aforementioned steps without any emotions.

If you remain calm, you will reduce power struggles and will have more success in shaping your child's obedient behavior. If it's getting "too hot" between you and your child, walk away, collect yourself, and wait until your child is calmer. Then go back and try again. See the "Staying Calm with a Stressful Child" section in Chapter 7 for more ideas on how to stay cool while interacting with your child.

Sometimes no matter how hard a parent tries, a heated argument ensues as the parent tries to get the child to comply with a command. **It is recommended that you discontinue removing privileges for disobedience if there is too much yelling or physical conflict.** Try another Success Plan in the book or consult a mental health professional about additional ideas to deal with the problem (see Chapter 10).

Step 5: Stay with It

The steps toward teaching your child to obey are effective only if you are **consistent and persistent.** Often, when these procedures fail, it is because the parent uses them only occasionally or gives up too easily. Be prepared, because it may take several weeks or months for a child to improve. Sometimes after a parent applies these procedures, a child's difficult behavior gets worse before it gets better. Don't be discouraged if this occurs. Try to avoid power struggles with your child and let your actions do the talking for you. Stay with it, and it will work. See Chapter 9 for more ideas on how to maintain improved behavior in yourself and your child.

Step 6: Practice with Charts

The **Time-Out** chart (at the end of this chapter) is for a preschool or early elementary school-age child (roughly 3–10 years old). Give it to him to inform and remind him of your expectation that he obey your commands and what will happen if he doesn't. The Time-Out chart can be copied and posted. Your child can refer to it when you tell him to do something, so he knows what will happen if he doesn't obey.

The **Removing Privileges for Disobedience** chart (at the end of this chapter) is for an older child/teen. As with the Time-Out chart, it informs and reminds the child/teen that parental commands need to be obeyed and what will happen if they are not. Your child/teen can refer to it when you tell him to do something, so he knows what will happen if he doesn't obey.

ACTIONS SPEAK LOUDER THAN WORDS

Back to Dan and Shelby: Dan decides to try some new and different approaches to working with Shelby. He realizes that "actions speak louder than words," and he decides to use the Time-Out procedure to improve Shelby's compliance. Dan is quick to praise Shelby when she is compliant with his commands or warnings, but whenever she "tests the limits" with disobedience, Dan is consistent in using Time-Out too. He noticed that Shelby needs to go in Time-Out less and less because she is more obedient. They are also arguing less. Dan is resolved to keep using these procedures.

CHILD SELF-CONTROL SUCCESS PLAN 2: TEACHING A CHILD TO FOLLOW RULES

WHEN WILL YOU EVER LEARN?

Harold and Opal have tried many times to get 13-year-old Jason to follow the household rules. Jason repeatedly doesn't do his homework, breaks his curfew, and sneaks out to the mall when he has been told not to go there. Harold and Opal are frustrated. They find themselves yelling at Jason a lot, which hasn't made much difference, because he still breaks the rules. Last night Harold was yet again yelling at Jason for coming in past curfew, and out of exasperation he asked Jason, "Will you ever learn?"

Discuss and Write Down the Rules

Many parents assume their child understands the rules, when in fact he may not. Sometimes parents have not explicitly stated what the rules are, or the child "forgets" or disregards them. It is helpful to communicate important rules clearly to your child.

Take some time by yourself to think of all the rules your child seems to violate. This might include not doing homework or chores, staying out too late, getting up too late in the morning, and so on. Write down all of the rules as a list and arrange the list of rules in order of importance. The most important rule would be on top and so forth. It is wise to focus on three or four of the most important rules as you begin. You can address other rules with your child at a later time.

Next, sit down with your child and **write down the rules on a piece of paper.** Be very clear and specific about the rules. For example, don't say, "Do your homework." Instead, say, "Do your homework each day before 7 P.M." Make sure your child clearly understands your rules. It may be helpful for each of you to have a written copy of the rules.

Then, on an occasional basis, **review the rules** and determine how well they are being followed by your child. The **Following the Rules** chart (at the end of this chapter) can be used to structure the rule-following evaluation process. Ask the child to look at each written rule and self-evaluate how well he thinks he has been following the rule over a specified period of time (e.g., day, week). Then give your child some feedback about how well you think he has been doing.

Be very careful about rules that restrict friendships. Sometimes if a parent restricts a child from a certain friend, the children find a way to see each other anyway. Although a parent can restrict friendships should he or she desire, it may be more successful to have **rules about friendships** instead. These rules might include stating where your child can go with the friend, a time to come home, and so forth. It may also be useful to get to know the other child's parents.

Establish and Enforce Daily Behavior Expectations

Discussing and writing down the rules is enough to improve many children's capacity to follow rules. If you think your child requires more work in this area, however, it may be useful to **recast the rules as daily behavior expectations and include rewards and punishments to improve behavior.** This section provides ideas on how to accomplish this and uses charts to organize the effort.

Step 1: Designate Behavior Expectations

Sit down with your child and discuss rules that are violated regularly. Often these are behaviors for which a parent frequently has to reprimand or remind a child to follow.

Examples of rules derived from problem behaviors might include:

- Complete chores or homework by a certain time.
- Go to bed at a certain time on school nights.
- Go to school each day.
- Feed the dog.
- Do not go to restricted areas (e.g., local mall or park) without permission.
- Do not go to a friend's home unless a parent is there.
- Tell a parent where you are going.

Step 2: Designate Privileges to Be Earned or Lost for Behavior

Discuss and specify extra privileges that your child can earn for following the rules and privileges your child can lose for not following the rules.

Examples of privileges to earn or lose might include the following:

- Using the phone
- Watching TV
- Using the car

- Being able to go outside
- Playing computer or video games

Step 3: Specify How Behavior Expectations Are Connected to Privileges

Write down the rules and behavior expectations, as well as privileges to be earned or lost on a chart (examples are discussed below). Thereafter, do not nag your child or remind him of rules and behavior expectations. Simply inform him of earned or lost privileges when he has or has not followed behavior expectations.

Different procedures should be considered for younger and older children. With a younger elementary school-age child, it is recommended that four or fewer behavior expectations be specified and that privileges be earned or lost each day. A day consists of a 24-hour interval determined by you (e.g., 6 P.M. Monday to 6 P.M. Tuesday). Review the rules with the younger child on a daily basis. With a more capable older elementary school-age child or teen, it is okay to have more than four behavior expectations and to give out rewards and consequences on a weekly basis.

Step 4: Practice with Charts

The **Daily Behavior Chart** (at the end of this chapter) can be used with **early elementary school-age children.** You'll note that the example chart provides visual feedback in the form of smiling and frowning faces to appeal to younger children. If you desire, your child can participate in drawing the smiling and frowning faces on the chart. Your child receives a small reward for doing one or two positive behaviors per day and a larger reward for doing three or four positive behaviors each day (see Appendix for more ideas on rewards and reinforcers for children). A negative consequence is only given if a child breaks all the rules for an entire day and receives all frowning faces. Review the chart on a daily basis. This means that your child's behavior is monitored over 1 day, and he receives reinforcement or consequences in accordance with the chart for 24 hours.

The **Weekly Behavior Chart** (at the end of this chapter) is for **late elementary school-age children and teens.** On this chart more behavior expectations can be added, and the behavior expectations are monitored on a weekly basis. Privileges are lost or earned based on a percentage of behavior expectations being followed that week and the corresponding "grade." It is still a good idea to review the older child's or teen's progress on a daily basis.

If you state the rules and episodically review them using the above procedures, your child will gradually come to "internalize" them. This means that the rules will become part of the child's memory, and he will recall them automatically when needed. Once your child has learned and internalized the rules, he will use them to guide his behavior without having to be reminded. The internalization of rules is an important step in developing self-control.

TEACHING A LESSON

Back to Harold, Opal, and Jason: Harold and Opal figured out that they could yell "until they turn blue" and it wouldn't help Jason follow their rules. They decided to try a Weekly Behavior Chart with him. Jason is not happy about the chart, but after losing some privileges for a few days for violating it, he begins to follow the rules better. Harold and Opal notice that Jason's behavior is improving and that they are arguing less with him.

CHILD SELF-CONTROL SUCCESS PLAN 3: TEACHING A CHILD TO MANAGE ANGER

BLOWING A CORK

Melissa is a 15-year-old who, according to her parents, Frank and Beverly, often "blows her cork." It takes very little to get her angry. Whenever things don't go her way or she gets frustrated, her parents expect her to explode with anger. Melissa seems to have this problem at home, at school, with her parents, and with her friends. It doesn't matter where she is or who she's with; she is prone to getting angry. Recently, because she could not find her jeans, she yelled at her mother. Another time Melissa became frustrated with her computer and threw the mouse across the room. If her parents confront Melissa about her behavior, she becomes even angrier. Although Melissa has never been violent, her parents are concerned that her anger problem might get worse.

Teaching Anger Management Skills

At the outset it is important to make sure your child has a true anger problem. **If your child is only angry when interacting with parents or family members, it may not be a real anger problem.** Instead, this behavior may be more about your child's disobedience, or it could be an indicator of family conflict. In these cases it may be wise to focus on the earlier sections of this chapter related to compliance and rule following or on the family conflict management strategies presented in Chapter 8.

When a child has habitual anger outbursts that seem out of proportion to the situation, and if it occurs in many settings such as home, school, or neighborhood, then it is a real problem that needs to be dealt with. The following section describes how you can help your child learn skills for handling anger. The intent is not to stop all angry feelings in a child, but for him to learn how to manage those strong feelings appropriately.

Step 1: Determine If Child Is Ready to Learn Anger Management Skills

Some children may not benefit from learning anger management skills because they are **too young or too resistant.** A young child (below the age of 8 to 10 years) may not have the reasoning abilities required to learn how to cope with anger on his own. Instead, teach a younger child how to understand and better express his feelings (see Chapter 5). Children can reduce anger outbursts if they learn how to put their feelings into words. Also, a child may be too defensive to learn how to cope with anger because he denies having an anger problem. In this case, emphasizing family conflict management may be more productive (see Chapter 8). Your child will be more cooperative if you show that everyone in the family is working on anger instead of just him. By participating in family conflict management training, your child will still be learning many skills that relate to anger management.

Step 2: Define Anger

You may be surprised to learn that many children with anger problems cannot accurately define anger! To be able to work on controlling anger, your child needs to understand what it is. Through a process of discussion with your child, come up with a definition of anger. Help your child understand that **anger is a feeling of discomfort or pain that occurs in response to something not going as one would like it to.** Explain to your child that angry feelings can range from frustrated (mild) to mad (moderate) to rage (severe). Ask your child to describe times or situations when he felt frustrated, mad, or rageful. Be sure to help your child define different levels of anger in future discussions of anger.

Step 3: Teach Child to Recognize Anger Signals

Learning to recognize when one is angry involves understanding the anger "signals." First explain that everyone feels anger, but it is how one handles it that determines whether or not it is a problem. Explain further that it is necessary to recognize when we are angry. Tell your child that just like a traffic light signals a driver about what to do at an intersection, anger also has three signals, including "body signals," "thought signals," and "action signals." Work with your child to develop a list on a piece of paper of all the body, thought, and action signals that you and he can generate.

Common body, thought, and action signals for anger are as follows:

Body signals
- Breathing rate increased
- Heart rate increased
- Sweating increased
- Red face color
- Tense muscles
- Body feels "hot."

Thought signals
- "I hate you."
- "I feel like telling her where to go."
- "You are so stupid."
- "I'm going to hit him."
- "I hate doing homework."
- "I want to break something."
- "I am dumb."
- "I can't do anything right."
- "I give up."

Action signals
- Punch/hit
- Yell
- Cry
- Threaten
- Faint
- Fidget
- Tremble
- Run
- Withdraw

After all of the signals have been listed, take some time to discuss and role play what these signals are all about. Ask your child to think about times when he was very upset and what signals he thinks may have applied during those situations. You could also discuss times when you were angry and the anger signals that applied to your situation. Your child and you could then physically demonstrate what the anger signals look like.

Step 4: Teach Child to Relax

Once your child has learned how to identify when he is angry, he then can then learn to control the anger. This is accomplished by **learning to reduce physical tension through relaxation.** The exact method for teaching a child to relax varies depending on the child's age.

The following is a list of possible methods you could use to instruct your child to relax:

- **Deep breathing.** Instruct, demonstrate, and have your child show how to do deep breathing exercises. The basic idea is to have him inhale deeply and exhale very slowly.
- **Visualization.** Have your child picture a very relaxing scene in his mind. For example, he might imagine himself floating on a raft on a lake. He would continue to visualize floating on the lake, going up and down gently with the waves, with the sun beating down, and so forth. Ask your child to identify his own personal visualization that he finds relaxing.
- **Robot/rag doll technique.** The robot/rag doll technique is a useful muscle tension/release relaxation approach used with younger children (age 10 years and below). At first, ask your child to tense up all the muscles in his body and visualize himself as a robot. Have him hold this tense state for approximately 15 seconds. Then ask him to release all the tension and visualize himself as a rag doll with all his muscles very loose. He should hold this relaxed state for 15 seconds. Have him continue to practice the robot/rag doll technique until he appears to know how to relax.
- **Systematic muscle tension/release relaxation procedure.** This procedure is better suited for older children and teens (age 11 and above). The basic idea is to have your child or teen tense up small muscle groups one at a time, starting at the lower end of the body and working up. For example, your child would tense up his feet, holding them tense for 5 to 10 seconds and then relaxing them for 5 to 10 seconds. This would be followed by going up to his lower legs, upper legs, abdomen, chest, shoulders, neck, and finally, the face. During each of these steps while he progressively goes up the body, he practices holding that particular area tense for 5 to 10 seconds, then releasing and maintaining a relaxed state for 5 to 10 seconds. Eventually, his entire body will be relaxed. Once your child becomes good at this, he can learn to relax all muscle groups simultaneously and quickly.

Try one or two of these methods over several meetings to teach your child to relax. Make sure he knows each skill before proceeding to the next skill.

Step 5: Teach Child to Use "Helpful Self-Talk"

This next skill involves talking to oneself in a helpful manner to calm down. First explain to your child that if he talks to himself in a helpful manner, he will be able to control anger better. Explain to your child that **helpful self-talk involves saying things to oneself (thoughts) to calm down.**

Below are examples of helpful self-talk:

- "Take it easy."
- "Stay cool."
- "Chill out."
- "Take some deep breaths."
- "I'm getting tense. Relax!"
- "Don't let him bug me."
- "I'm going to be OK."

- "It's OK if I'm not good at this."
- "I'm sad Tanya doesn't want to play with me, but many other kids like to play with me."
- "I'll just try my hardest."
- "Try not to give up."

After your child seems to understand the purpose of helpful self-talk, then you can move on to demonstration and role-play exercises. You could demonstrate how to use helpful self-talk when you are angry. For example, you could get frustrated with trying to fix the plumbing under the kitchen sink. First, you could demonstrate a poor way to handle this particular situation (e.g., throwing tools, swearing, and yelling). Next you could show how to manage this same situation better utilizing helpful self-talk such as, "I need to relax," "I'm going to cool down," "I won't let this get to me," and so forth. After you have demonstrated this skill several times, ask your child to do similar role plays.

Step 6: Teach Child to Take Action

The final step in learning how to manage anger is to take action and/or solve the problem that originally made the person angry. **Taking action might involve expressing feelings, asking for a hug, going for a walk, relaxing, being assertive with someone, and so forth.** Problem-solving skills, which are discussed in Chapter 4, can also be used to take action. It is important to tell your child that he still needs to solve the problem that made him feel upset. Review all the procedures with your child so that he understands what taking action is all about.

Step 7: Practice with Charts

One method of helping a child apply these new skills in everyday situations would be simply to ask him to use the skills when needed. If your child becomes angry or frustrated, you might say something like, "This is a good time to practice cooling down." The **Cool Down** chart (at the end of this chapter) can be used as a visual cue to guide your child through the steps of anger management. You might remind your child to look at this chart as he is trying to cool down. Be sure to notice, comment, and praise your child for using the skills. Try to reinforce your child regularly and often enough to promote his use of the skills.

A structured procedure for helping your child use the anger-coping skills involves completing the **Anger Management Worksheet** (at the end of this chapter). Ask your child to complete this worksheet when he gets angry. Your child can fill out this chart either independently or with your guidance, depending on what you think is best for him. It's not that important who actually completes the chart, just that it be used to structure the anger-coping process. If desired, a reward could be given to the child for positive ratings on the Anger Management Worksheet. See the Appendix for more ideas on rewards for children.

CAPPING THE CORK

Back to Melissa, Frank, and Beverly: Frank and Beverly decide that they are going to try to take some action with young Melissa. They sit down with her at a time when the family is relaxed. They explain how Melissa can learn how to control her anger with anger management skills. At first Melissa is resistant, but through a friendly and supportive discussion, they get her to acknowledge that she may benefit from working on anger management skills. They go through all the steps and procedures for learning to recognize when one is angry, as well as learning how to cope with feelings of anger through relaxing, using helpful self-talk, and taking action. Melissa and her parents have worked out an agreement that when she is able to use the Anger Management Worksheet successfully five times, she will have earned the privilege of going to a concert of her choice. At first Melissa stumbles and has difficulty. At one point her mother asked her to use anger coping, and that made her even angrier. Gradually, however, Melissa began to incorporate the anger management strategies. At this point she still gets angry occasionally, but her anger outbursts have become less frequent, and she is aware of her anger problem.

CHARTS FOR CHAPTER 3

TIME-OUT

1.

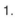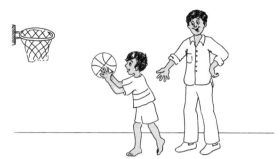

Command—if . . . then: "I want you to. . . ."

2.

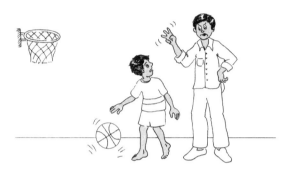

Warning—if . . . then: *If* you don't [command], *then* you will have to go to time out.

3.

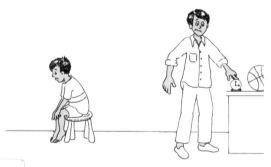

Time-Out—sit in chair and set timer.

TIME-OUT

1. 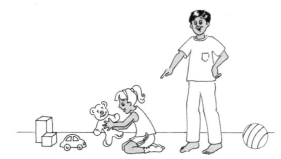 **Command**—if . . . then: "I want you to. . . ."

2. 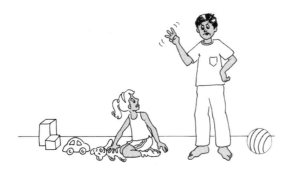 **Warning**—if . . . then: *If* you don't [command], *then* you will have to go to time out.

3. 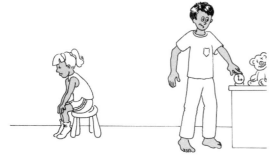 **Time-Out**—sit in chair and set timer.

TIME-OUT

1. 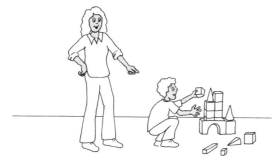 **Command**—if . . . then: "I want you to. . . ."

2. 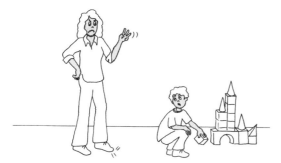 **Warning**—if . . . then: *If* you don't [command], *then* you will have to go to time out.

3. 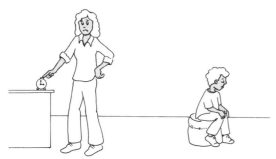 **Time-Out**—sit in chair and set timer.

TIME-OUT

1. 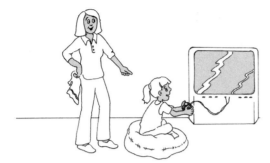 **Command**—if . . . then: "I want you to. . . ."

2. 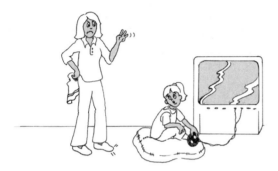 **Warning**—if . . . then: *If* you don't [command], *then* you will have to go to time out.

3. 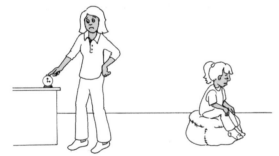 **Time-Out**—sit in chair and set timer.

REMOVING PRIVILEGES FOR DISOBEDIENCE

1. **Parent states a command to child/teen.** The command should be brief and clear as to exactly what is expected of the child/teen.

2. **Give a warning.** If the child/teen does not follow through with the command, then the child/teen should be given a warning. A warning is an **"if . . . then"** statement. The warning should be stated clearly and concisely. For example, "If you don't [command], then [you will lose a privilege]." Privileges to remove may include TV time, access to the telephone, going outside, driving, games, and so forth. It may be helpful to count to 3 before going to the next step.

3. **Loss of privilege.**

   Option 1: The child/teen is told that the privilege is lost until he/she complies with the original command.

   Option 2: The child/teen is told the privilege is lost for a specified period of time (e.g., 24 hours).

4. **After compliance.** Once the child/teen has complied with the original command, the lost privilege is returned in accordance with Option 1 or 2 above.

FOLLOWING THE RULES

1. I think I was following the rules . . .

2. You think I was following the rules . . .

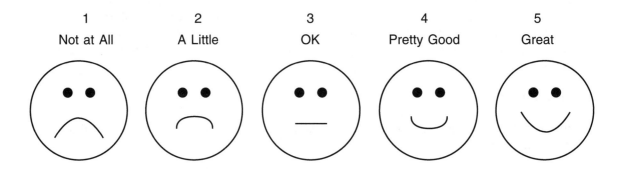

1	2	3	4	5
Not at All	A Little	OK	Pretty Good	Great

EXAMPLE: DAILY BEHAVIOR CHART

Name: _April_

Week of: _November 6–12_

Directions: Identify four (or fewer) target behaviors for your child to work on each day. Put a smiling face in the box if the behavior was completed. Put a frowning face in the box if the behavior was not completed. Always praise your child for a smiling face. At the end of the day, tally up smiling and frowning faces. Administer the reward or mild punishment sometime within 24 hours. There are two levels of reward and one level of mild punishment.

Behavior	Mon.	Tues.	Wed.	Thur.	Fri.	Sat.	Sun.
Up and dressed by 7:00 A.M.	☹	☺	☹	☺	☺		
Homework done before supper	☹	☺	☹	☺	☺		
Take dog out for walk	☹	☹	☺	☺	☺		
In bed by 7:30 P.M. with lights out	☹	☺	☺	☺	☺		

	Mon.	Tues.	Wed.	Thur.	Fri.	Sat.	Sun.
Total smiling faces	0	3	2	4	4		
Total frowning faces	4	1	2	0	0		

Daily reward:

1–2 Smiling faces = _Snack_

3–4 Smiling faces = _Rent favorite DVD_

Mild punishment:

4 Frowning faces = _No computer for 24 hours_

DAILY BEHAVIOR CHART

Name: _____

Week of: _____

Directions: Identify four (or fewer) target behaviors for your child to work on each day. Put a smiling face in the box if the behavior was completed. Put a frowning face in the box if the behavior was not completed. Always praise your child for a smiling face. At the end of the day, tally up smiling and frowning faces. Administer the reward or mild punishment sometime within 24 hours. There are two levels of reward and one level of mild punishment.

Behavior	Mon.	Tues.	Wed.	Thurs.	Fri.	Sat.	Sun.

	Mon.	Tues.	Wed.	Thurs.	Fri.	Sat.	Sun.
Total smiling faces							
Total frowning faces							

Daily reward:

1–2 Smiling faces =

3–4 Smiling faces =

Mild punishment:

4 Frowning faces =

EXAMPLE: WEEKLY BEHAVIOR CHART

Week of: _____

Name: _____

Behavior	Saturday	Sunday	Monday	Tuesday	Wednesday	Thursday	Friday
Help with dishes	√	√		√	√	√	
Bathroom cleanup after shower		√	√	√	√	√	√
Write in school planner	N/A	N/A	√	√			√
Cooperate with good attitude around the house	√	√	√	√	√		√
Ask for permission to use Internet	√	√	√		√	√	√
Come home on time (9:00 P.M. on school nights and 11:00 P.M. on weekends)		√	√	√	√		

Weekly Grade and Corresponding Rewards/Consequences (Determined on <u>Friday Evening</u>   )

A = 36–40 (90%)—$10 and stay up late two weekend nights or sleep over

B = 32–35 (80%)—$7 and stay up late one weekend night

C = 28–31 (70%)—$5

F = < 27 (< 69%)—grounded all weekend

WEEKLY BEHAVIOR CHART

Week of: _____

Name: _____

Behavior	Saturday	Sunday	Monday	Tuesday	Wednesday	Thursday	Friday

Weekly Grade and Corresponding Rewards/Consequences (Determined on _____)

A =   (90%)—

B =   (80%)—

C =   (70%)—

F =   (< 69%)—

COOL DOWN

1. Am I angry?

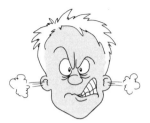

2. Cool down my body.

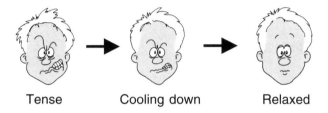

Tense   Cooling down   Relaxed

3. Use cool-down thoughts.

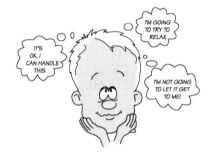

4. Do something to solve the problem.

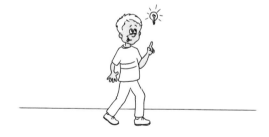

COOL DOWN

1. Am I angry?

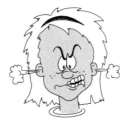

2. Cool down my body.

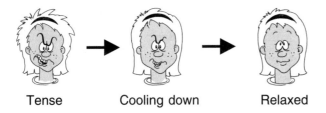

Tense   Cooling down   Relaxed

3. Use cool-down thoughts.

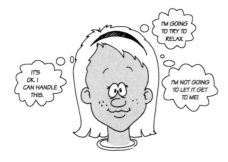

4. Do something to solve the problem.

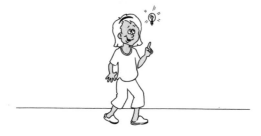

EXAMPLE: ANGER MANAGEMENT WORKSHEET

Name: _Melissa_

Date: _Sunday_

Directions: A child and/or parent can complete this worksheet. It's best to fill out the worksheet while you are angry, but it's also OK to fill it out afterward.

1. **What event or problem is making me feel angry?**
   The kid next door keeps bugging my friends and me. He won't leave us alone.

2. **What are the signals that tell me I am angry?**
   a. **Body signals:** My muscles are tense. My heart is pounding.
   b. **Thought signals:** I wish he would go away. He's going to steal my friends.
   c. **Action signals:** I yelled at him.

3. **What can I do to relax my body?**
   I will take some deep breaths and try to relax my body.

4. **What "helpful self-talk" can I use to control my thoughts?**
   "Don't let him bug me." "Keep cool." "Relax."

5. **What effective action can I take to deal with the situation or solve the problem?**
   I'll talk to him. I'll ask him to let me play with my friends alone. If that doesn't work, I'll ask Dad for help.

Anger Management Rating (circle one)

1. Didn't try anger management at all.
2. Sort of tried anger management, but it didn't really work.
3. Tried hard with anger management, but it didn't really work.
4. Tried hard with anger management, and it worked.

ANGER MANAGEMENT WORKSHEET

Name: _____

Date: _____

Directions: A child and/or parent can complete this worksheet. It's best to fill out the worksheet while you are angry, but it's also OK to fill it out afterward.

1. **What event or problem is making me feel angry?**

2. **What are the signals that tell me I am angry?**
   a. **Body signals:**
   b. **Thought signals:**
   c. **Action signals:**

3. **What can I do to relax my body?**

4. **What "helpful self-talk" can I use to control my thoughts?**

5. **What effective action can I take to deal with the situation or solve the problem?**

Anger Management Rating (circle one)

1. Didn't try anger management at all.
2. Sort of tried anger management, but it didn't really work.
3. Tried hard with anger management, but it didn't really work.
4. Tried hard with anger management and it worked.

Chapter 4

Enhancing a Child's Social Development

Social problems in struggling children often originate from negative social behaviors the child emits such as interrupting, bossing, poor eye contact, fighting, and difficulty solving everyday social problems that occur between people. Children who struggle in the social arena are prone to be rejected by positive-influence peers and then either become withdrawn or hang out with children who get in trouble. To be successful, a child must learn to use positive social behaviors while interacting with others and develop the ability to solve social problems.

This chapter provides three Child Social Success Plans for parents to encourage social development in their struggling child:

Child Social Success Plan 1: Teaching a Child Social Behavior Skills— provides information on how to teach a child positive social behaviors such as sharing, taking a turn, and so on (see pages 76–80).

Child Social Success Plan 2: Teaching a Child Social Problem-Solving Skills—shows how to teach a child to resolve social problems in a step-by-step manner (see pages 81–87).

Child Social Success Plan 3: Promoting Positive Peer Affiliations— encourages a child's associations with positive-influence peers (see pages 87–89).

Each of these three Child Social Success Plans works better with children at different developmental stages. Social behavior skills training in Child Social

Success Plan 1 is a good place to start with a younger child or an older child/ teen who has not yet learned these important behaviors. Since social problem solving involves sophisticated reasoning abilities, not all children can benefit from this type of skill development. Therefore it is recommended that only a child who is at least 8–10 years old be exposed to social problem-solving skills training as described in Child Social Success Plan 2. Encouraging positive peer influences as described in Child Social Success Plan 3 is a good idea for children of all ages but is especially relevant for teens, given the amount of time they spend with peers. Review Chapter 2 for additional information if you are uncertain of your child's level of social development.

It is important to note that early parent–child relationships and family interactions have a lot to do with children's ultimate social skills. Therefore, if a family is stressed out, a parent might want to examine the family skills training information presented in Chapter 8 prior to working on the child's social development or perhaps at the same time.

CHILD SOCIAL SUCCESS PLAN 1: TEACHING A CHILD SOCIAL BEHAVIOR SKILLS

NOBODY LIKES ME

Tony is a 10-year-old boy with few friends. At a recent school conference, Tony's teacher told Debbie and Bruce that their son bugs other children and gets into fights with kids. At home, Debbie and Bruce notice similar problems between Tony and his 8-year-old sister, Kathy, as well as with other children in the neighborhood. They are concerned because Tony seems to be picked on, teased, and rejected by other children. Although Tony often plays with children in the neighborhood and does OK at first, after a little while it's not uncommon for Tony to come home crying, "Nobody likes me."

Social Behavior Skills Training

Many children who have difficulty in getting along with others exhibit too many negative social behaviors, such as hitting, interrupting, or bugging, and too few positive social behaviors, such as making eye contact, expressing feelings, or cooperating. If your child does not typically employ positive social behavior skills in social situations, she may need to have them taught to her. This section describes how parents can teach a child to develop social behavior skills.

Step 1: Identify Social Behaviors to Target

Below is a list of social behaviors you can focus on with your child. The first task is to figure out which negative social behaviors your child displays too often and which positive social behaviors your child does not employ often enough.

Examples of negative social behaviors include the following:

- Physical aggression
- Playing unfair
- Arguing
- Interrupting
- Name calling
- Bossing others
- Whining, complaining, and so forth
- Taking others' possessions
- Dominating the activity
- Making poor eye contact
- Being a poor sport
- Being too loud
- Showing off
- Teasing
- Butting in
- Bugging others
- Getting into others' space
- Withdrawing and isolating self
- Letting others be too bossy
- Poor listening
- Hoarding food, toys, etc.
- Keeping feelings inside
- Talking too much
- Disobeying rules of play
- Being too rough in play
- Succumbing to peer pressure

Examples of positive social behaviors include the following:

- Taking turns
- Sharing
- Expressing feelings
- Cooperating
- Making eye contact
- Starting conversations
- Being assertive
- Listening to others
- Complimenting others
- Accepting compliments
- Following rules of play
- Sticking up for oneself
- Apologizing to others
- Asking questions
- Telling others about self
- Playing fair
- Ignoring when appropriate
- Inquiring about others' interests
- Talking in a brief manner
- Asking for what one wants/needs
- Helping others
- Inviting others to do something
- Refusing to participate in negative activities with peers

To figure out which social behaviors to focus on with your child, it will be helpful to take time to observe her in social situations with peers and/or siblings. To get the information you need, it may be necessary to watch your child for several days or weeks in various social situations. You should observe your child in situations that are highly structured, such as scouting events, sports, and church activities, and those that are unstructured, such as playing with peers or siblings in the front yard or at the park. Try to notice if your child is accepted by her peers. Note whether your child seems to be rejected or neglected, or is aggressive or bullies other children. Furthermore, watch for negative social behaviors your child displays too often and positive social behaviors your child doesn't use enough (see previous examples of negative and positive social behaviors). After you have observed your child and thought about it, select one or two negative social behaviors to reduce and one or two positive social behaviors to increase in your child.

Step 2: Work with Child in Selecting Target Social Behavior(s)

It is very important to **collaborate with your child** in selecting and working on specific positive social behaviors. This is sometimes a delicate situation because some children are nervous or defensive about working on social behaviors. At first, try to discuss the problem with your child in a supportive manner. Begin by pointing out that she seems to have some difficulty getting along with other children. Don't judge your child, but communicate to her that you would like to help. Explain that you have a plan for how she might be able to get along better with other children and that you would like to work with her to put this plan into action. **Don't bother trying to work with your child regarding social behavior skills until this cooperative parent–child relationship has been achieved.**

Next, review a list of possible negative and positive behaviors (such as in the previous section). Ask for your child's input about which negative social behaviors she thinks she should do less and which positive social behaviors she thinks she should do more. If you think it would be helpful, share your observations regarding her interactions with other children. Together, select a target positive social behavior. Ideally the positive social behavior selected will be the opposite of a negative social behavior of your child's (e.g., sharing instead of hoarding or taking turns instead of being bossy).

Step 3: Teach Child to Perform the Positive Social Behavior(s)

This step involves teaching your child to perform physically the selected positive social behavior skills. First, explain each targeted positive social behavior in a way she will understand. Then demonstrate what the behavior looks like. Next role play the behavior by taking turns acting it out until your child can demonstrate the behavior. Usually, after explaining, demonstrating, and role playing most children have a good understanding of the targeted behavior. For example, if your child is working on starting conversations, explain what starting conversations is all about, demonstrate what it looks like to start conversations, and then have the child practice starting conversations through role playing. **Make sure your child completely understands and is able physically to perform the targeted social behavior before going on to the next step.**

Step 4: Coach and Reward Desirable Social Behaviors in Social Situations

Coaching is critical in helping a child use a newly acquired social behavior skill in real-life situations. **Coaching involves prompting or reminding your child to be aware of and physically to perform positive social behaviors.** You can coach your child to practice the social behavior skills in everyday parent–child, sibling–child, or peer–child interactions. All of these social interactions provide good opportunities to practice social behavior skills. It might also be helpful to plan ahead about how your child could work on a social behavior skill in future social situations. For example, if a parent knows that a child will be going to her cousin's birthday party, the parent and child might plan ways for the child to work on a social behavior during the party. For example, a parent could state, "Remember to work on sharing when you go to your cousin Jamie's party today at Aunt Sue's house." In this example, when your family goes to the birthday party, you would remind your child to share.

Rewarding social behavior can be done in a formal or informal manner. Formal rewarding involves giving your child a tangible reward for practicing the desired social behavior, such as a toy or extra privilege. See the Appendix for more ideas on rewards for children. The informal reward procedure is accomplished by verbally praising your child when she engages in the desired social behavior.

Step 5: Hang in There

Social problems in children are difficult to change. It can take weeks, months, or even years for a child to use a new skill on a regular basis. Even if your child changes her behavior, others still may not change their opinion of your child due to previous labeling. For these reasons, you may need to work a long time to improve your child's social behavior. It's going to take time to help your child develop social behavior skills and be accepted by other children.

Step 6: Practice with Chart

The **Daily Social Behavior Goals** chart (at the end of the chapter) can be used to help your child practice social behavior skills. The chart requires that you or your child write down one or more social behaviors she will work on that day. At the end of the day, your child rates herself using the 5-point scale found on the chart to evaluate how well she met her social goal(s). You also rate your child on how well she met the social goal(s) and provide reinforcement if she did a good job. If your child receives ratings of 3 or more on the chart, she could earn a reward (see Appendix for more suggestions on rewards and reinforcers for children). The Daily Social Behavior Goals chart can be used to improve social behaviors in parent–child, sibling–child, and peer–child interactions.

SOMEBODY LIKES ME

Back to Tony: His parents, Debbie and Bruce, decide they need to help Tony develop social behavior skills. At first, they observe Tony at play in the neighborhood, at his little league baseball practice, and with his sister, Kathy. They observe that Tony seems isolated at first, then gradually interacts more and more negatively with other children. He interrupts, bosses, and bugs the other kids and very rarely takes turns or shares. It appears as though Tony is unaware that he is bothering other children.

Later, Debbie and Bruce talk to Tony and enlist his cooperation, and he agrees to work on sharing and taking turns. They explain what sharing and taking turns is, demonstrate what sharing and taking turns looks like, and then engage Tony in role plays where he shows example behaviors of sharing and taking turns. The role plays continue until Tony can physically demonstrate what sharing and taking turns looks like. They make use of the Daily Social Behavior Goals chart, first focusing on Tony sharing and taking turns with his sister and then with other children in the neighborhood. Gradually Tony's social behavior improves, and he earns rewards for his efforts. Debbie and Bruce are pleasantly surprised when Tony is invited to a classmate's overnight birthday party.

CHILD SOCIAL SUCCESS PLAN 2: TEACHING A CHILD SOCIAL PROBLEM-SOLVING SKILLS

WHY DON'T YOU THINK ABOUT WHAT YOU'RE DOING?

Sally is 14 years old and is seemingly always in trouble. Her mother, Brenda, frequently has to discipline Sally for her misbehavior. Brenda can cite numerous incidents when Sally didn't think about what she was doing. For example, she recently told Sally to rake up some leaves in the front yard. When a friend came by on her bike, Sally put down her rake and went off to the park with her. This type of behavior grew worse when a friend talked Sally into stealing some candy from a local convenience store and they both got caught by the store clerk. Similar difficulties also occur at home. Recently Sally's younger brother, Michael, changed the channel on the TV from a show that Sally was watching. Sally's immediate response was to punch Michael. Brenda is tired of yelling at Sally and punishing her for this kind of behavior. She frequently asks Sally, "Why don't you think about what you're doing?"

Social Problem-Solving Training

Social problem-solving training is especially useful for children who have a track record of disagreements with peers. This type of training is designed to help children learn to recognize social problems, think of alternative strategies and consequences, anticipate obstacles, and apply effective tactics to solve social dilemmas. Parents can assist their child in learning these important skills by following the steps below.

Step 1: Determine If Child Can Benefit from Social Problem-Solving Training

Children of all ages can benefit to varying degrees from training in social problem solving. But social problem-solving skills require sophisticated thinking ability. **It may be difficult for children under the age of 8–10 to apply social problem-solving strategies in real-life situations very well because they do not think in abstract terms.** Children over age 8–10 are developmentally more ready and can benefit to a greater extent from social problem-solving training. These older children are also more likely to apply the strategies on their own.

Parents should not expect a child to use social problem solving if she does not typically obey instructions or follow rules or if she cannot control anger. **If your child is frequently disobedient, routinely breaks the rules, or is often too angry, don't try to teach her social problem solving until those problems are addressed.** You will have more success with a focus on enhancing your child's obedience, rule following, or anger management as discussed in Chapter 3 first. Perhaps after your child is more agreeable, better at following rules, and can control anger better, then you could teach her social problem solving.

Step 2: Collaborate with Child

You won't get too far in teaching your child social problem-solving skills without her cooperation. Therefore, it is necessary to take some time to discuss the purpose and goals of social problem solving. Explain that social problem solving helps a child make and keep friends, get along with siblings, and so on. Don't blame or point fingers, but instead focus on the future and how social problem solving can help her get along with others. **Make sure your child is willing to work with you before working on social problem-solving skills.** It is absolutely critical that your child understand her difficulty in solving social problems and is ready to learn.

Step 3: Instruct Child in Social Problem Solving

Review the **Social Problem Solving** chart (at the end of the chapter). You will likely need to discuss and demonstrate how to use each social problem-solving step as portrayed in the chart. **Start with easy social problems and then apply the skills with more difficult social situations.** While discussing the social problem-solving steps, it may be helpful to present a made-up social problem and ask your child questions to lead her to solve it. For example, you might ask your child to solve the social problem that comes up when she wants to watch a certain TV show, but her brother wants to watch a different one. Continue instructing your child in this manner and guide her to solve as many made-up social problems as needed until she understands what social problem solving is all about.

An important point to keep in mind is that many children have a very difficult time with Step 6 of the Social Problem Solving chart (i.e., do the plan). This requires performing a specific behavior to solve the problem. **Just because a child thinks of a good plan (e.g., "I'll ignore him") doesn't mean she can actually do the plan (e.g., actually ignore him).** Many children need to be taught how to do the plan (e.g., taught how to ignore). This can be accomplished by instructing, demonstrating, and practicing specific social behaviors as described in Child Social Success Plan 1 in this chapter.

Step 4: Instruct Child in Situation Interpretation and Perspective Taking

Some children make mistakes in how they interpret other people's intent in social situations and do not think of others' points of view. Situation interpretation and perspective-taking training helps a child accurately judge social situations and think of others' viewpoints more accurately. These skills require a child to think about her own thoughts in order to evaluate their accuracy and to think of others' perspectives. Since situation interpretation and perspective-taking training requires abstract thinking abilities, **this type of training is recommended for children over 10 years old.**

Situation interpretation training helps your child understand how different people see or understand problems differently. For example, in baseball, an umpire might call a base runner out at home, while the runner may think she is safe. Another example is a child who is bumped by another child while walking down the hall. She might think the other child bumped her on purpose. Another child might think she was bumped by accident. Discuss other examples of how people differ in how they see situations and sometimes make mistakes. Ask your child to think of times when she made mistakes in interpreting others' behavior.

Explain that people can stop and figure out if they are seeing situations correctly or not. For example, an NFL football receiver catches a pass but is called out of bounds by a referee. The football receiver and his coach think he was in bounds and protest the referee's call. The referee could ask another referee for a second opinion or review the videotape to make sure he called the play correctly. After this process of checking it out, the referee might change his original call. Explain that the same can be true of social situations. A person might be bumped in the hallway, think the person who bumped her did it on purpose, but after thinking about it could change her mind to think it was an accident. Ask your child to look for the evidence as to who caused a problem. The evidence includes, but is not limited to, thinking about the other person's facial expression, how the other person behaved after the episode, etc. Explain that looking for evidence is the key to seeing "sticky situations" accurately. Tell your child that when something happens to her, it is important to stop and think, "Who or what caused the problem?"

Perspective-taking training helps your child put herself in the other person's shoes, to understand others' thoughts and feelings. As a starting point, you could page through a magazine, look at pictures, and ask your child to think of each person's thoughts and feelings. Next ask your child to reflect on past, real-life social situations she was involved in that didn't go too well. For example, your child may recall taking a toy from a friend or sibling yesterday. Again, ask your child to try to explain what she and the other person were thinking and feeling. Tell your child that when something happens to her, it is important to stop and think, "What does each person think and feel?"

Try to incorporate discussions of situation interpretation and perspective taking into ongoing social problem-solving discussions. The Social Problem Solving chart incorporates these two skills. **Step 2—Who or what caused the social problem?—is designed to focus a child on interpreting situations accurately.** As you discuss Step 2 with your child, ask her to state her role and the other person's role in creating the problem. **Step 3—What does each person think and feel?—is designed to focus a child on understanding others' perspectives.** As you discuss Step 3 with your child, ask her to state what she thinks are the thoughts and feelings of each person who is involved in a particular social problem.

Step 5: Demonstrate Social Problem Solving

You can be a better teacher by demonstrating social problem solving to your child. For example, talk out loud about problems such as what to make for dinner, plans for the evening, where to go out to eat, and so forth. Later, demonstrate use of problem-solving strategies for increasingly difficult problems, such as how to deal with a difficult boss at work, minor problems with a friend, and so forth. It is recommended that you **avoid discussing adult-only personal problems** (e.g., marital or financial problems) with your child to demonstrate how to solve problems.

You could demonstrate use of the problem-solving steps in either a formal or an informal manner. A formal way of modeling problem solving involves referring to the Social Problem Solving chart. You could have this chart in hand and go through each step as you solve a problem, while your child observes. Problem solving can also be demonstrated in an informal way by thinking through situations and problems out loud for your child to observe. For example, when confronted with a problem, you could say something like, "Hmm, I wonder what the problem is here. What should I do? I think I will try (a strategy/plan). Did it work?" and so forth.

Step 6: Assist Child in Using Problem Solving through "Guided Questioning"

Try to facilitate your child's application of social problem solving in real-life situations by asking guided questions in either a forced-choice or open-ended manner. For a younger child, or an older child who gets "stuck" and can't come up with the answer, the forced-choice method could be used. The older child or teen who possesses a few more skills in this area can benefit from open-ended guiding questioning.

Examples of forced-choice guided questions include the following:

1. "You could try this (option 1) or that (option 2). What do you think would work best?"
2. "It looks like you have two options. This (option 1) or that (option 2). What do you think would work best?"

Examples of open-ended guided questions include the following:

1. "What can you do?"
2. "I am confused. Explain it to me. How could you solve that problem?"
3. "How are you going to solve that problem?"
4. "What's the first step? Then what do you do? OK, now what's the next step?"

Don't solve your child's problems for her. Try to help your child solve her own problems through guided questions. For example, if your child complains that she cannot get along with a friend, don't suggest what she can do; instead prompt her to use the problem-solving process to figure it out for herself.

Step 7: Practice with Charts or Worksheets

The Social Problem Solving chart (at the end of the chapter) can be used to guide a child through the social problem-solving steps. Look at the chart together as you guide her to solve a particular social problem. Each time your child or teen solves a social problem, you should praise her for the hard work.

A structured method of practicing social problem solving involves using the **Social Problem-Solving Worksheet** (at the end of the chapter). This worksheet can be used to solve immediate social problems or to think retroactively about how social problems could have been solved. **Act as a coach and**

guide your child in the social problem-solving process by using the worksheet. After you and your child have worked through a Social Problem-Solving Worksheet, the last step is to evaluate your child as to how well she used the social problem-solving procedure. A 4-point rating scale can be found at the bottom of the worksheet. Its purpose is to give your child some feedback about how well she used social problem solving. To motivate your child you may want to provide a reward for completion of the charts and for obtaining ratings of 3 or 4 (see the Appendix for more ideas on how to reward children).

You or your child could fill out the Social Problem-Solving Worksheet. It's not so important who actually writes on the worksheet, but that it is used as a vehicle to structure the social problem-solving process. You could act as the "secretary" and write down what your child says if that makes your child more willing to use the procedure.

Family Problem Solving

The procedures described above are designed for child-focused social problem solving. **Using child-focused social problem solving, however, implies that the child has the problem, and some children are defensive about this implication.** Family problem solving involves solving problems between family members. **Family problem solving sometimes works better than child-focused social problem solving.** Younger children (under age 8–10) and some teens (who don't like to be singled out) often prefer and benefit more from the family problem-solving approach. See Chapter 8 for more details on family problem solving.

THINKING BEFORE ACTING

Back to Sally and Brenda: Brenda decides that she's going to try to teach Sally to "think before she acts" through social problem-solving training. After Brenda teaches Sally the social problem-solving process, she guides Sally to apply it with the aid of the Social Problem Solving chart. At first, they practice solving social problems pertaining to minor disagreements between Sally and her brother. Later Sally is encouraged to use the Social Problem-Solving Worksheet after a social problem occurred with a friend. Brenda worked out a deal with Sally where she can earn a new music CD for using five Problem-Solving Worksheets. Gradually, Sally began to use the social problem-solving process on her own. Brenda was startled one day when Sally actually came up to her and said, "Mom, I think I'm going to use a Social Problem-Solving Worksheet to solve a problem I am having with Michael." Sally has continued to show progress in learning the social problem-solving technique.

CHILD SOCIAL SUCCESS PLAN 3: PROMOTING POSITIVE PEER AFFILIATIONS

THE "WRONG CROWD"

Herbert is baffled as to why his 15-year-old son Rodney is getting into so much trouble at school and in the neighborhood. Herbert has received phone calls from school about Rodney wandering the halls and smoking cigarettes with friends in the parking lot. Although his curfew is 11:00 P.M., last Saturday Rodney waltzed in at 12:30 A.M., smelling of alcohol. The last straw was when the police brought Rodney home because he was caught throwing apples at cars with some of his friends. It seems that all Rodney wants to do these days is hang out with his friends and roam the neighborhood. Herbert is concerned that Rodney is going to end up getting into serious trouble because he is hanging out with the "wrong crowd."

Research has demonstrated that peers have a large influence on a child's development and that if a child hangs out with kids who get in trouble, she has increased odds of getting in trouble herself. Even as early as preschool and early elementary school it has been shown that aggressive children tend to associate together. In the teen years, those who skip school, use drugs, and engage in risky behavior tend to join together. The reverse is true too. Kids who are well-adjusted and stay out of trouble tend to associate with each other. In short, it appears that "birds of a feather flock together," and that these birds exert considerable influence!

In view of this information, it makes sense to promote positive peer affiliations in your child. The overarching idea is to orchestrate and arrange for your child to be with positive-influence peers. Below are some common-sense ideas to make this happen.

Teach Child Social Skills

Children with poor social skills are more likely to end up rejected by positive-influence peers. They bug, annoy, hit, spread rumors, and so on, which does not bode well for making and keeping friends. These rejected children are vulnerable to negative-influence peers. If you teach your child social behavior and social problem-solving skills like those in this chapter, she will be better able to make and keep friends.

Get Child Involved with Positive Organizations and Institutions

Positive-influence peers are found in organizations and institutions that provide structured and goal-oriented activities. Churches, community centers, schools, and park and recreation boards provide scouts, organized sports, after-school programs, arts and music activities, and other similar programs. These places and the activities they provide facilitate a positive peer culture, and many encourage parents to participate or lead activities. Children who are involved in such organizations and activities have opportunities to form friendships with positive-influence peers, and they learn from observing positive peer role models.

Monitor Peer Activities

Get to know your child's friends and be aware of what they are doing. Make an effort to talk to your child's friends and inquire about their interests. Try to make your home an inviting place that has fun activities for your child and her friends. It is also advised to make connections with the parents of your child's friends and coordinate efforts in keeping track of them. **When your child or teen goes out always discuss the "4 W's."** This entails explicitly stating rules and limits regarding (1) Where she is going, (2) Who she'll be with, (3) What she'll be doing, and (4) When she'll be home. The 4 W's provide parameters and boundaries regarding the child or teen's social activities. All of these monitoring strategies will give you information about your child's friends and what they are up to so you can minimize the impact of negative-influence peers.

THE "RIGHT CROWD"

Back to Rodney and his father Herbert: Herbert can see the writing on the wall, and he aims to stop Rodney from getting into any further trouble. He knows that Rodney is being influenced in a negative way by his current group of friends. Herbert recalls how much Rodney used to love playing baseball, but for some reason he dropped out of it a few years back. Herbert talks Rodney into rejoining a baseball team, and he volunteers to be an assistant coach. They end up spending a lot of time together on the baseball diamond, and Rodney becomes friends with some of his new teammates. Herbert seizes the opportunity and invites Rodney and his new friends to play pool on the new pool table he just bought for the basement. Now when Rodney is away from the house, Herbert always knows the 4 W's, and for the most part, Rodney has been cooperating. It seems Rodney is on a better track now that he is affiliating more with positive-influence peers.

CHARTS FOR CHAPTER 4

EXAMPLE: DAILY SOCIAL BEHAVIOR GOALS

Name: _Tony_

Date: _Saturday_

Directions: Indicate below which positive social behavior goals you will be working on. At the end of the day, rate how well you accomplished your goals. It may be helpful to get feedback from parents as to how well they think you are accomplishing your goals.

Child Evaluation

1. **I am working on these social behavior goals:**
   Sharing and expressing feelings.

2. **How well did I accomplish my goals?** (circle one)

1	2	3	(4)	5
Not at all	A little	OK	Pretty Good	Great

Parent Evaluation

3. **How well parent thinks child accomplished social behavior goals:** (circle one)

1	2	3	(4)	5
Not at all	A little	OK	Pretty Good	Great

Reward

4. **If my parent rates me as a 3,4, or 5, I get this reward:**
   Pizza for supper.

DAILY SOCIAL BEHAVIOR GOALS

Name: _____

Date: _____

Directions: Indicate below which positive social behavior goals you will be working on. At the end of the day, rate how well you accomplished your goals. It may be helpful to get feedback from parents as to how well they think you are accomplishing your goals.

Child Evaluation

1. **I am working on these social behavior goals:**

2. **How well did I accomplish my goals?** (circle one)

1	2	3	4	5
Not at all	A little	OK	Pretty Good	Great

Parent Evaluation

3. **How well parent thinks child accomplished social behavior goals:** (circle one)

1	2	3	4	5
Not at all	A little	OK	Pretty Good	Great

Reward

4. **If my parent rates me as a 3, 4, or 5, I get this reward:**

SOCIAL PROBLEM SOLVING

1. **Stop! What is the social problem?**

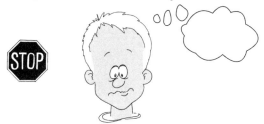

2. **Who or what caused the social problem?**

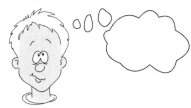

3. **What does each person think and feel?**

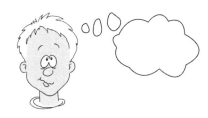

4. **What are some plans?**

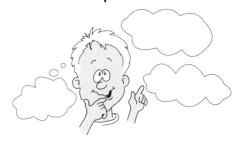

5. **What is the best plan?**

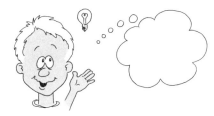

6. **Do the plan.**

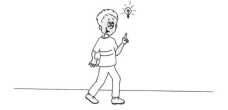

7. **Did the plan work?**

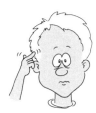
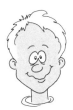

SOCIAL PROBLEM SOLVING

1. **Stop! What is the social problem?**

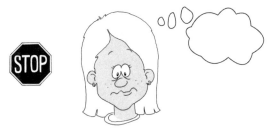

2. **Who or what caused the social problem?**

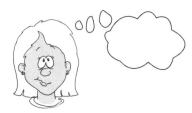

3. **What does each person think and feel?**

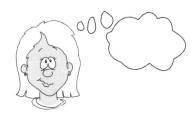

4. **What are some plans?**

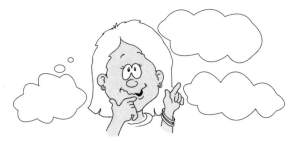

5. **What is the best plan?**

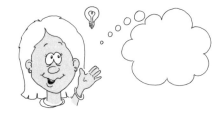

6. **Do the plan.**

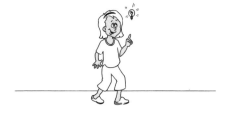

7. **Did the plan work?**

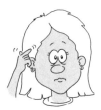 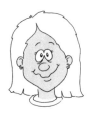

EXAMPLE: SOCIAL PROBLEM-SOLVING WORKSHEET

Name: _Sally_

Date: _Tuesday_

Directions: The parent and/or child can complete this form. You can use the worksheet to solve a social problem as it occurs or to figure out how you could have solved a social problem after it's over.

1. **Stop! What is the social problem?**

   I want to watch a show on TV, but my brother wants to watch a different show.

2. **Who or what caused the social problem?** (optional) Try to figure out your role and other people's roles in causing the social problem.

   We both have a role in this social problem because we want to watch different shows.

3. **What does each person think and feel?** (optional) Put yourself in the "other guy's shoes" to see how that person thinks and feels.

   My brother and I both want to watch our own show, and we both feel frustrated.

4. **What are some plans (solutions)?** List as many plans (solutions) as possible that could be used to solve the social problem.

   I could watch my show. He could watch his show. I could ask Mom to help. We could try to work out a deal.

5. **What is the best plan?** Think ahead about what would happen if you used the plans in Step 4. Then decide which one will work best.

   I will try to work out a deal with my brother.

6. **Do the plan.** How will I do the plan? What will I do to make the plan work?

   I will ask my brother if we could take turns. I will ask him to watch my show now, and we can watch a show he wants next.

7. **Did the plan work?**

   He said OK. It worked.

Social Problem-Solving Rating (circle one)

1. Didn't use social problem solving at all.
2. Tried to use social problem solving a little, but it didn't really work.
3. Tried hard, went through social problem-solving steps, but didn't really use the best plan.
4. Tried hard, went through social problem-solving steps, and used the best plan.

SOCIAL PROBLEM-SOLVING WORKSHEET

Name: _____

Date: _____

Directions: The parent and/or child can complete this form. You can use the worksheet to solve a social problem as it occurs or to figure out how you could have solved a social problem after it's over.

1. **Stop! What is the social problem?**

2. **Who or what caused the social problem?** (optional) Try to figure out your role and other people's roles in causing the social problem.

3. **What does each person think and feel?** (optional) Put yourself in the "other guy's shoes" to see how that person thinks and feels.

4. **What are some plans (solutions)?** List as many plans (solutions) as possible that could be used to solve the social problem.

5. **What is the best plan?** Think ahead about what would happen if you used the plans In Step 4. Then decide which one will work best.

6. **Do the plan.** How will I do the plan? What will I do to make the plan work?

7. **Did the plan work?**

Social Problem-Solving Rating (circle one)

1. Didn't use social problem solving at all.
2. Tried to use social problem solving a little, but it didn't really work.
3. Tried hard, went through social problem-solving steps, but didn't really use the best plan.
4. Tried hard, went through social problem-solving steps, and used the best plan.

From *Skills Training for Children with Behavior Problems: A Parent and Practitioner Guidebook* (revised edition) by Michael L. Bloomquist. Copyright 2006 by The Guilford Press. Permission to photocopy this chart is granted to purchasers of this book for personal or professional use only (see copyright page for details).

Chapter 5

Enhancing a Child's Emotional Development

Some struggling children keep their feelings inside, think unhelpful thoughts that make them feel bad, and end up suffering from low self-esteem. Unfortunately these children can develop additional emotional difficulties such as depression or anxiety, and because they feel bad inside, may be prone to act out through defiance, aggression, or other emotional outbursts. Such children would benefit from learning to express everyday feelings, think helpful thoughts about self and others, and develop a positive sense of self-esteem.

This chapter presents three Child Emotional Success Plans that parents can use to teach their child emotional skills:

Child Emotional Success Plan 1: Teaching a Child to Understand and Express Feelings—assists a child learn to be more aware of and express feelings through words (see pages 100–103).

Child Emotional Success Plan 2: Teaching a Child to Think Helpful Thoughts—helps a child learn to identify and change unhelpful thoughts to helpful thoughts (see pages 103–106).

Child Emotional Success Plan 3: Promoting a Child's Self-Esteem—presents common-sense approaches that parents can employ to boost the self-esteem of children at all ages (see pages 106–110).

Each of these different Child Emotional Success Plans can be used with children of different ages. Child Emotional Success Plan 1, learning to understand and express feelings, is especially useful for a younger child or an older child/teen who did not learn those important skills early on. Since "thinking about thoughts" is a task requiring complex reasoning, the helpful thinking skills outlined in Child Emotional Success Plan 2 are primarily for older children and teens. The self-esteem boosters presented in Child Emotional Success Plan 3 apply to children of all ages.

It needs to be pointed out that emotional development is closely related to self-control development and, in particular, managing strong emotions such as anger. Therefore, if a parent is intent on building a child's emotional skills, it may be wise to also work with the child in the area of anger management skills as described in Chapter 3.

CHILD EMOTIONAL SUCCESS PLAN 1: TEACHING A CHILD TO UNDERSTAND AND EXPRESS FEELINGS

WHAT'S GOING ON IN THERE?

Eleven-year-old Dominique has always been more defiant and aggressive than most kids. His parents, Keisha and Willie, often have to deal with angry outbursts and tantrums. Over the past several months Dominique appears increasingly sad and withdrawn. He rarely discusses his problems or feelings. Sometimes Keisha is concerned and asks Dominique, "What's going on in there?"

Feelings Education and Expression Training

A number of struggling children have a very narrow range of emotional experience. Some of them are angry most of the time, while others are nervous or sad. They have a hard time understanding their own feelings, let alone expressing them. Parents can teach their child about their own feelings and how to express them appropriately.

Step 1: Increase Child's "Feelings Vocabulary"

If your child does not have a feeling word in his vocabulary, he cannot express that particular emotion very well. For example, if your child does not understand or use the word "enraged," he may not be able to express himself adequately when he is extremely angry and upset. Instead of saying what he feels, he may *act out* his emotions.

The first step in helping your child increase his feelings vocabulary is to instruct him about different feelings. The **Feelings Vocabulary Chart** (at the end of the chapter) can be used for this purpose. This chart lists a variety of feeling words, with accompanying facial expressions. Show the chart to your child. Ask your child if he understands all the words on the chart. Ask him if he has experienced any of the feelings shown on the chart. If you are unsure how to explain a particular feeling word, you may want to look up the word in the dictionary. It's important to explain the words clearly so that your child understands each feeling shown on the chart. With younger children, you may want to circle 10 "basic" feelings to focus on instead of the whole list.

It might be helpful to discuss and role play different situations that create certain feelings. For example, someone sleeping in bed at night who is awakened by a loud noise might feel "frightened." Try to get your child actively involved in discussing situations that might bring about different feelings.

Step 2: Demonstrate the Expression of Feelings

One extremely powerful way children learn how to express feelings is by observing their parents. If a parent keeps his or her feelings inside, the child may deal with emotions in a similar way. **If a child observes a parent expressing feelings regularly, that child will be more likely to do so as well.**

Try to be aware of times when you are experiencing feelings and express them. Practice expressing these feelings so that your child can observe your demonstration. This can be done in a formal or informal manner. Expressing feelings in a formal manner might involve experiencing an emotion, getting out the Feelings Vocabulary Chart, pointing to a facial expression, and using the word on the chart to express a feeling. For example, if you burn some food on the stove, you could get out the chart, point to the feeling of frustrated, and state that you are feeling "frustrated." Expressing feelings in an informal way can be accomplished simply by talking out loud while you are experiencing emotions. For example, if you burn something on the stove, you would simply state out loud, "Boy, that makes me feel frustrated."

Step 3: Practice Being Aware of and Expressing Feelings

A good method to practice expressing feelings involves routinely discussing feelings and the events that elicit them each day. Ask your child to express himself when you see him experiencing an emotion, such as when your child is upset because you told him to shut off the TV and do homework. You might use this opportunity to ask him to express his feelings. Prompting can take the form of asking open-ended questions such as "What are you feeling right now?" or a closed question such as "Are you angry?" Sometimes it is necessary to be persistent and supportive when trying to assist a child to express feelings. Keep asking questions and offer support until the child expresses the feeling. **If your child becomes too upset at your questions, drop it and try again another time.**

A final way you can help your child understand his emotions is to label feelings for him. This can be especially helpful for a younger child or when a child is either defensive or unwilling to participate in a discussion of feelings. For example, you might notice your child is upset when you tell him to shut off the TV and do homework and simply state, "You look angry." Look for opportunities to discuss and label your child's feelings as events unfold.

You can reinforce your child in an informal way simply by praising him when he expresses feelings. When your child does express his feelings, you might state, "I'm proud of you for expressing your feelings," "I'm glad you expressed your feelings to me," "You did a good job expressing your feelings," and so forth.

Step 4: Practice with Chart

One method to help your child practice being aware of expressing feelings involves using the **Feelings Diary** (at the end of the chapter). The Feelings Diary requires your child to write down positive and negative events that occur in his daily experience and the feelings that accompany these events.

The child should have the option of sharing the diary or keeping it private. Many children also benefit when a parent fills out a Feelings Diary and shares it with the child. This helps the child feel less alone in the process and gives the child the added benefit of learning by observing the parent. If you decide to keep a Feelings Diary too, be sure to write about neutral and not-too-personal events. For example, it would be helpful to write about how you felt in a traffic jam, but not how you felt while arguing with your spouse or partner.

LET'S TALK ABOUT IT

Back to Dominique, Keisha, and Willie: One day Dominique comes home from school and goes straight to his room and shuts the door. Willie follows Dominique and knocks. Dominique lets his father in the room. Dominique looks sad, but he won't say what is going on. Because Willie is persistent, Dominique gradually talks about being teased by some kids at school. At first he blames the kids and looks angry, but eventually Dominique admits he feels sad. Willie praises Dominique for talking about his feelings and says he will try to help Dominique any way he can.

Later Willie proposes that he and Dominique try to work on expressing their feelings. They review the Feelings Vocabulary Chart. They discuss and role play different feelings. Willie shows Dominique the Feelings Diary. He suggests that he and Dominique tell Keisha about this and that all three of them use it to work on understanding and expressing feelings. Dominique agrees to this plan. After using these charts for a week, Willie notices that all three family members are using more feelings words in their everyday conversation and that Dominique seems less sad.

CHILD EMOTIONAL SUCCESS PLAN 2: TEACHING A CHILD TO THINK HELPFUL THOUGHTS

I'M SO STUPID

Thirteen-year-old Jennifer has had a tough year. She gets in trouble about two or three times a week at school. Although Jennifer has several friends around the neighborhood, other kids at school tease her. At home, she and her single father, Jeff, argue a lot. Jeff thinks they have more negative interactions than positive ones. Over the year, Jennifer has become increasingly irritable and moody. Sometimes she comes home from school, slams the door, and stomps her feet. When Jeff asks, "What's wrong?" Jennifer responds loudly and abruptly, "Nothing!" Jennifer has also been watching more TV lately. She just doesn't seem very happy.

Yesterday Jeff received Jennifer's report card in the mail and noticed several poor grades. That evening Jeff asked Jennifer to explain why some of her grades were low. Jennifer replied, "Because I'm so stupid!"

Changing Unhelpful Thinking

This section is designed to give parents ideas on how to help older children (age 10 and up) change negative or unhelpful thinking patterns. This is accomplished by helping a child identify unhelpful thoughts, understand the unhelpful nature of these thoughts, and change the thoughts to be more help-ful. If your child can learn these important helpful thinking skills, he will experience more positive emotions.

Step 1: Determine If Child Is Ready to Learn to Change Unhelpful Thinking

Children under the age of 10 may not yet have the mental abilities to profit from this approach. Also, children who have not yet acquired the ability to understand and express feelings, regardless of their age, may not be able to accomplish the skills outlined in this section. If your child is too young or has not mastered the skills of understanding and expressing feelings, it may be more productive to first focus on Child Emotional Success Plan 1.

You will need to have a series of discussions with your child to work on changing unhelpful thoughts. Be sure that your child is a willing participant in these discussions. Do not force your child to do this. **If your child is resistant, take the time to discuss your concerns about him in a supportive manner to enlist his cooperation. If that does not work, then perhaps some of the skills discussed elsewhere in this book should be emphasized instead of this approach.**

Step 2: Identify Unhelpful Thinking

Unhelpful thinking involves thinking thoughts that are untrue, blown out of proportion, magnified, "awfulized," or otherwise negative. **Explain that a person's thought influences his feelings and behavior.** For example, if your child attempts to give a piano recital and thinks, "I'm going to do awful," "I'm too nervous," and so forth, then he will feel nervous and might perform poorly. However, if he is giving a piano recital and thinks, "I'll do the best I can" or "If I try, I'll do fine," he will feel more confident and likely perform well. Discuss other examples until your child sees a relationship among thoughts, feelings, and behavior.

Next ask your child to do self-evaluation by completing the **Unhelpful Thoughts for Children** chart (at the end of the chapter). Guide your child to complete the chart and ratings accurately. If you think it would help the dis-cussion, you could also complete the same chart and rate how you believe your child thinks (i.e., the parent rates the child on a separate chart). At the end of the Unhelpful Thoughts for Children chart are several questions. Ask the child to answer those questions for thoughts rated as a 3. The goal is for your child to recognize that his thoughts may be making him feel bad and that they are not helping his situation. Using this chart as a springboard, continue to discuss how negative thinking is often unhelpful.

Step 3: Change Unhelpful Thinking

The next task is to teach your child to counter unhelpful thinking with helpful thinking. To accomplish this, you can use the **Helpful Thoughts for Children** chart (at the end of the chapter) in conjunction with the Unhelpful Thoughts for Children chart. Thought #1 on the Unhelpful chart can be countered (or replaced) with Thought #1 on the Helpful chart and so on. There are more questions at the end of the Helpful chart to ask for each thought. Guide your child to answer these questions about his own helpful thoughts. The goal now is for your child to recognize that helpful thoughts may make him feel better and that these thoughts may help his situation. Ideally your child will see the benefit of these helpful thoughts.

Step 4: Demonstrate Helpful Thinking

One powerful method to help your child learn how to think in a more helpful way is for you to demonstrate this type of thinking for him. As discussed elsewhere in this book, children learn a lot by observing their parents. **They may learn a "good way" or a "bad way" to think based on their observations of you.**

One way to demonstrate helpful thinking is simply to talk out loud when you notice that you are thinking unhelpful thoughts. For example, you might try to patch up some cement work in the basement and not do a very good job. You might make some disparaging comments such as, "This looks terrible! I can't do anything around the house. I must be all thumbs." Then you might say something such as, "This is unhelpful thinking. I'm going to try to change my thoughts. Just because I can't do cement work very well doesn't mean the world is going to end or that I'm a terrible person. It would be more helpful to realize that I can't do everything perfectly, and, even if I did mess up, it's not the end of the world."

Step 5: Practice with Charts or Worksheet

The **Helpful Thinking** chart (at the end of the chapter) can be used as a visual aid for changing thoughts. You might want to remind your child to look at this chart as he is trying to change his thoughts. Be sure to notice, comment, and praise your child for using this skill.

The **Changing Unhelpful Thoughts Worksheet** (at the end of the chapter) can be used to help your child apply these skills in real life. This chart can be completed either on the spot or after a problem has occurred. Prompting a child to use helpful thinking skills can be done by noticing when the child may be thinking an unhelpful thought (as evidenced by what the child says) and asking him to change those thoughts. Questions such as, "Are you sure that thought is helpful?" or "Are you thinking in a helpful way?" would suffice. When you notice your child doing unhelpful thinking, you could ask him to use helpful thinking and then praise him if he does so. Another way to encourage helpful thinking is to provide a reward to your child for completing a set number of Changing Unhelpful Thoughts Worksheets. See the Appendix for more ideas on rewards for children.

I GUESS I'M OK

Back to Jeff and Jennifer: Jeff's concern about Jennifer culminated in him deciding to try to help her think more positively. He realized that both he and Jennifer are "negative thinkers." Jeff introduces the notion of trying to change unhelpful thinking to Jennifer one day when she is in a good mood. They have several discussions about unhelpful thinking. Jeff makes a point to demonstrate helpful thinking and to discuss informally what's happening when he thinks in an unhelpful manner around the house. Jennifer and Jeff both fill out Changing Unhelpful Thoughts Worksheets for several weeks. Jeff tells Jennifer that he will buy her that new purse she has been asking for if she successfully completes five worksheets. On one recent occasion, Jeff observed Jennifer talking about changing her thoughts without any prompting. Jennifer seems happier since they have been working on increasing helpful thinking.

CHILD EMOTIONAL SUCCESS PLAN 3: PROMOTING A CHILD'S SELF-ESTEEM

WHAT'S WRONG WITH YOU?

Eight-year-old Marcus lives with his parents, Sharon and David, and his 6-year-old sister, Stacy. Marcus has a long history of behavior problems, including being defiant with his parents and being aggressive with his sister and some of the neighborhood children. Sharon and David have had countless arguments with Marcus over the years, and sometimes they argue with each other about what to do with him. Several parents in the neighborhood complain about Marcus, which increases the tension between Marcus and his parents.

Sharon and David try to be as positive as they can but often find themselves saying negative things to Marcus when they are angry and upset with him. A typical example of this occurred the other day when Marcus grabbed some of Stacy's toys from her and ran. Stacy became very upset and ran after Marcus, and a big argument developed in Marcus's room. David came into the room to find his two children screaming at each other. He had heard what had gone on prior to this, and he knew that Marcus was in the wrong. He was so steamed up and angry that he shouted at Marcus, "What's wrong with you?"

Common-Sense Ideas to Promote Self-Esteem

Parents play a vital role in promoting a child's self-esteem. Although heredity has much to do with determining who we are, the role of parents is also critically important. Parents can have a profound influence on their child's development of positive self-esteem by using some of the suggestions below.

Give Positive Feedback

What parents say and how they say it has a great impact on their child's self-esteem. During childhood, a child receives feedback from others—the most important feedback coming from parents. If the negative feedback outweighs the positive feedback, the child will develop a negative view of self. **If the positive feedback outweighs the negative feedback, over time the child will develop a positive view of self.** Providing more positive feedback than negative feedback is quite challenging for parents of a struggling child. Look for small good things your child does and praise him for these successes. Spend less time correcting your child and more time reminding him of what he does well.

Be Involved

For a child really to feel good about himself, he has to know that his parents care about him and are involved in his life. Some of the ideas described in Chapter 8 of this book help increase parent involvement. **Try to improve the quality of your relationship with your child by becoming more involved in his everyday life.**

Maintain Healthy Family Interactions

Everyday family interactions have a strong effect on a child. Pay attention to and emphasize the family interaction skills discussed in Chapter 8. In particular, **try to avoid certain kinds of communication such as negative questions, blaming, putdowns, and sarcasm** (see Chapter 8 for more details). A negative style of communication will dampen a child's self-esteem. If a child repeatedly hears negative statements about himself, it is likely he will see himself as bad. **Good communication and problem solving within the family will promote your child's self-esteem.**

Really Listen

It is very tempting to correct your child or give him advice in regard to his troubles or difficulties. This can turn your child off. He may avoid talking to you. **Really listening to your child can help him feel better about you and himself.**

There are several methods you can use to improve listening. One method is paraphrasing. This involves restating what your child says so that he knows you really understand him. Another method is to accept your child's feelings (even if you disagree with his behavior). Tell the child what you think he feels like or restate the feeling he expresses.

Be Accepting

Many of a struggling child's problems are chronic and very difficult to change. It may not be useful to keep focusing on the same problem(s) over and over. **Try to determine which behaviors you can realistically change and which behaviors you need to accept.**

Handling Mistakes and Failures

A child with behavioral or adjustment problems tends to make many mistakes and sometimes feels like a failure. The child may struggle at school, have fewer friends, get in trouble, or say things he shouldn't. When a problem arises do not "shame" your child by dwelling on it or asking, "Why did you do that?" Instead give your child a consequence, if needed, and **ask what he can learn from this mistake.** Also, try to downplay your child's mistakes (e.g., a low grade on a test). Assure him it's OK. Tell him that the main thing is to keep trying. Then help him focus on effort (trying) rather than outcome (success or failure).

Accepting Successes

A child with low self-esteem sometimes does not like to admit he did something good. Doing something good doesn't fit with his self-concept. For example, if a child with low self-esteem does well on a test, he may minimize his responsibility for that good grade. If a child with low self-esteem has a success, he may think it was because he was lucky, or it was too easy, or someone else is responsible. When your child does something well, help him see that he is responsible for his successes. Remind him that if he works hard he can do well.

Promote Talents

Every child has a talent, whether it is in art, sports, music, dance, working with animals, volunteer work, or fixing computers. **Make an extra effort to help your child develop whatever talent he has.** Your child will be able to receive more positive feedback from honing his talents, thus raising his self-esteem.

Don't Attribute Good Behavior to Medications

Some struggling children who have psychiatric disorders such as ADHD, depression, or anxiety are taking prescribed medications. Sometimes a parent will make the mistake of asking the child if he "took the pill" when he misbehaves. Sometimes a parent will describe a child's positive behavior as resulting from taking the medication. Over time this can have a negative effect on a child's self-esteem. He may begin to think that he is not a good person unless he is on medication.

If your child is taking medication and is one of those who show a positive response, make sure you don't put too much emphasis on the effects of the medication when your child is behaving well. Even if medication is having a positive effect on your child, be sure and help him see that he is the one responsible for his positive behavior.

Teach Developmental Skills

Parents can teach a child important life skills to become successful. If a child is successful, he will receive more positive feedback from others and will feel good about himself. **Try to work on helping your child develop the skills described in this book because they will help him succeed, which will ultimately enhance his self-esteem.**

ACCENTUATE THE POSITIVE

Back to Marcus, David, Sharon, and Stacy: David and Sharon are concerned about Marcus's self-esteem. They realize that the way they have been talking to Marcus and dealing with some of his behaviors has been too negative and may be contributing to his low self-esteem. They are now determined to "accentuate the positive" with Marcus. They decide to teach him how to understand, identify, and express his feelings. They resolve to give him much more positive feedback and to try to accept him more for who he is. After several weeks they notice that they are indeed being more supportive and positive, not only to Marcus, but to Stacy and to each other. They hope that if they continue to emphasize the positive, Marcus's self-esteem will improve.

CHARTS FOR CHAPTER 5

FEELINGS VOCABULARY CHART

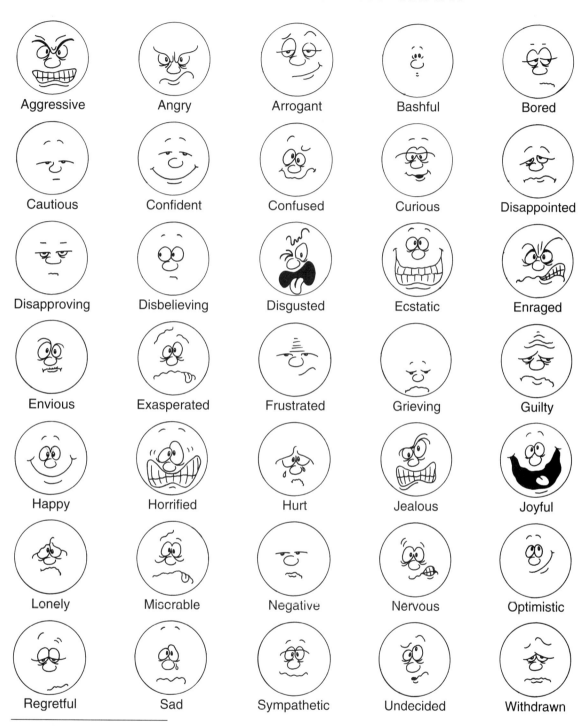

Aggressive	Angry	Arrogant	Bashful	Bored
Cautious	Confident	Confused	Curious	Disappointed
Disapproving	Disbelieving	Disgusted	Ecstatic	Enraged
Envious	Exasperated	Frustrated	Grieving	Guilty
Happy	Horrified	Hurt	Jealous	Joyful
Lonely	Miserable	Negative	Nervous	Optimistic
Regretful	Sad	Sympathetic	Undecided	Withdrawn

EXAMPLE: FEELINGS DIARY

Name: Dominique

Date: Friday

Directions: Write down positive and negative events that happened to you. Then write down how you felt in response to those events. Use the Feelings Vocabulary Chart to help you label your feelings. You can fill the diary out when an event occurs or afterward. You can share this Feelings Diary with others or keep it private.

Positive Events

1. I got a star on my math worksheet.

2. My mom hugged me.

3.

4.

My Feelings

1. Happy

2. Happy, joyful

3.

4.

Negative Events

1. Joe pushed me.

2. Some kids called me names.

3.

4.

My Feelings

1. Mad, sad

2. Lonely, scared

3.

4.

FEELINGS DIARY

Name: _____

Date: _____

Directions: Write down positive and negative events that happened to you. Then write down how you felt in response to those events. Use the Feelings Vocabulary Chart to help you label your feelings. You can fill the diary out when an event occurs or afterward. You can share this Feelings Diary with others or keep it private.

Positive Events   **My Feelings**

1.   1.

2.   2.

3.   3.

4.   4.

Negative Events   **My Feelings**

1.   1.

2.   2.

3.   3.

4.   4.

UNHELPFUL THOUGHTS FOR CHILDREN

Listed below is a variety of thoughts children may have about themselves. Read each thought and indicate how frequently that thought (or a similar thought) typically occurs for you over an average week. There are no right or wrong answers to these questions. Ask for help if you don't understand something on this form. Use the 3-point rating scale to answer how often you have these thoughts:

1	2	3
Rarely	Sometimes	Often

Thoughts about Self

1. ____ I'm no good.
2. ____ I can't do anything right; I'm a failure.
3. ____ I'm a brat.
4. ____ I have to do well in school, sports, and so forth, or people will look down on me.

Thoughts about Peers

5. ____ Most of the kids don't like me.
6. ____ Most of the kids think I'm stupid.
7. ____ Most of the kids think I'm a pest.
8. ____ I don't fit in with the crowd.

Thoughts about Parents/Family

9. ____ Our family is all messed up.
10. ____ It's my fault the family is having problems.
11. ____ My parent is to blame for my problems at home.
12. ____ My parent wants to run my life.
13. ____ My parent is unfair.

Thoughts about Teacher/School

14. ____ The teacher is to blame for my problems at school.
15. ____ My teacher is unfair.
16. ____ I give up. It's no use trying at school anymore.

(continued)

Thoughts about the Future

17. ____ My future doesn't look good. I see trouble ahead.

18. ____ I give up. I've tried everything. There's nothing more I can do.

For each thought you rated a 3, ask yourself the following questions:

1. What is unhelpful about this thought?
2. How does this unhelpful thought make me feel?
3. Is it a good idea to keep thinking this thought?

HELPFUL THOUGHTS FOR CHILDREN

Listed below are helpful "counter" thoughts that children can use instead of unhelpful thoughts. Unhelpful Thought #1 corresponds to Helpful Thought #1 and so on. Compare the unhelpful thoughts to the helpful thoughts.

Thoughts about Self

1. I'm too hard on myself. I'm OK.
2. I make mistakes, but I also do a lot of things OK.
3. I can behave positively too.
4. All I can do is keep trying. I have to accept myself for who I am. I'll concentrate on what I do well.

Thoughts about Peers

5. It's impossible for everyone to like me. Some of the kids do like me.
6. I'm blowing it out of proportion. Some of the kids think I'm OK.
7. I'm blowing it out of proportion. Some of the kids think I'm OK.
8. I fit in with some people. I do have friends.

Thoughts about Parents/Family

9. It doesn't help to think about the family being all messed up. Instead we need to take action.
10. It's not all my fault. Other people also play a role in the problems.
11. It doesn't help to blame my parent. I should focus on solutions to the problems.
12. My parent is trying to help. If I would take more responsibility, my parent would probably let up on me.
13. My parent seems unfair at times, but if I really look at it, I know that my parent treats me OK.

Thoughts about Teacher/School

14. It doesn't help to blame my teacher. I need to think about solutions.
15. My teacher is trying to help. If I would take more responsibility, my teacher would probably let up on me.
16. It doesn't help to give up. I need to keep trying.

(continued)

Thoughts about the Future

17. I'm being irrational. I have no proof that I will have problems in the future. I need to wait until the future.
18. I can't give up. I have to keep trying.

For each countering thought you choose, ask yourself the following questions:

1. What is helpful about this thought?
2. How does this helpful thought make me feel?
3. Is it a good idea to keep thinking this thought?

HELPFUL THINKING

1. Am I thinking unhelpful thoughts?

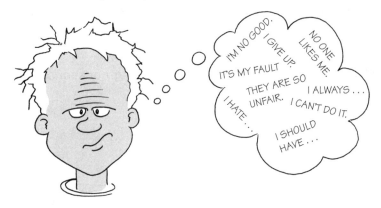

2. Are these thoughts going to help me?

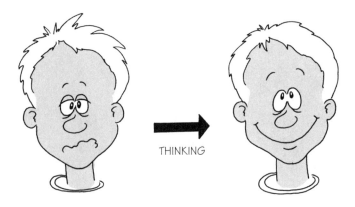

3. What is a different or more helpful way I can think?

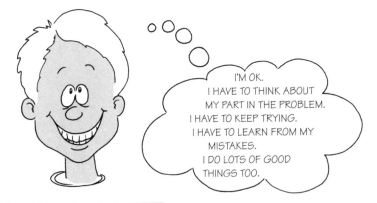

HELPFUL THINKING

1. Am I thinking unhelpful thoughts?

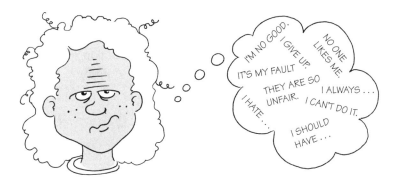

2. Are these thoughts going to help me?

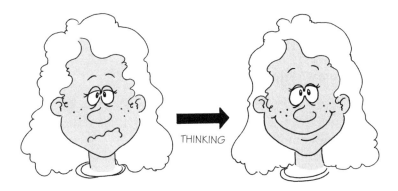

3. What is a different or more helpful way I can think?

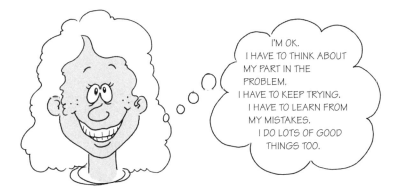

EXAMPLE:
CHANGING UNHELPFUL THOUGHTS WORKSHEET

Name: Jennifer

Date: Tuesday

Directions: A child and/or parent can complete this worksheet. Answer each question as it pertains to changing unhelpful thoughts. Fill out the worksheet during or after you have experienced an unhelpful thought.

1. **Am I thinking unhelpful thoughts?**
   Yes

2. **What is the unhelpful thought I am thinking?**
   Sarah doesn't like me.

3. **How do my unhelpful thoughts make me feel?**
   Awful, sad, lonely.

4. **Is it helpful to keep thinking this thought?** Why or why not?
   No. It makes me feel sad.

5. **What is a different or more helpful way I can think?**
   Sarah probably does like me. I might be imagining that she doesn't. We usually play together. It doesn't help me to think this thought.

6. **How does the new helpful thought make me feel?**
   Better. I feel happier.

7. **Is it helpful to keep thinking the new thought?** Why or why not?
   Yes. I'll try to play with Sarah more often.

Changing Unhelpful Thoughts Rating (circle one)

1. Didn't change my thoughts to be more helpful at all.
2. Tried a little to change my thoughts to be more helpful, but it didn't really work.
3. Tried hard, went through the steps, but it didn't help to change my thoughts.
4. Tried hard, went through the steps, and changed my thoughts to be more helpful.

CHANGING UNHELPFUL THOUGHTS WORKSHEET

Name: _____

Date: _____

Directions: A child and/or parent can complete this worksheet. Answer each question as it pertains to changing unhelpful thoughts. Fill out the worksheet during or after you have experienced an unhelpful thought.

1. **Am I thinking unhelpful thoughts?**

2. **What is the unhelpful thought I am thinking?**

3. **How do my unhelpful thoughts make me feel?**

4. **Is it helpful to keep thinking this thought?** Why or why not?

5. **What is a different or more helpful way I can think?**

6. **How does the new helpful thought make me feel?**

7. **Is it helpful to keep thinking the new thought?** Why or why not?

Changing Unhelpful Thoughts Rating (circle one)

1. Didn't change my thoughts to be more helpful at all.
2. Tried a little to change my thoughts to be more helpful, but it didn't really work.
3. Tried hard, went through the steps, but it didn't help to change my thoughts.
4. Tried hard, went through the steps, and changed my thoughts to be more helpful.

Chapter 6

Enhancing a Child's Academic Development

Children who struggle in the academic arena display their difficulties in many ways, including off-task behavior, poor organizational skills, incomplete assignments, and delays in academic subjects (reading, math, written language), to name but a few. Unfortunately many struggling children fall farther and farther behind at school. Some of them become so frustrated they give up and act out as a way of coping with failure. At its worst, when they get older, some struggling children drop out of school. If a child's academic development can be facilitated, she may be able to avoid problems and increase the odds of academic success.

This chapter provides three Child Academic Success Plans for parents to use to improve their child's academic abilities including:

Child Academic Success Plan 1: Helping a Child Appreciate and Enjoy Reading—suggests ways parents can promote a positive attitude about reading in their children (see pages 126–128).

Child Academic Success Plan 2: Teaching a Child Self-Directed Academic Behavior Skills—focuses on the everyday behaviors that children need to employ to be successful at school including organization, study skills, and staying on task (see pages 128–133).

Child Academic Success Plan 3: Being Involved in a Child's Schooling—presents ideas and strategies to be an active participant in a child's school experience (see pages 133–135).

These Child Academic Success Plans may be more relevant to children at one age versus another. Typically younger children enjoy the suggested activities found in Child Academic Success Plan 1 to promote a positive attitude toward reading. Children in the early elementary grades and up benefit from instruction on developing self-directed academic behavior skills as described in Child Academic Success Plan 2. The ideas for enhancing parent involvement in a child's schooling, as detailed in Child Academic Success Plan 3, are good for youth of all ages.

Of course some children may struggle at school in spite of being excited about reading and having good self-directed academic behaviors and involved parents. These struggling children may have learning or behavioral disorders that get in the way of their achievement at school. It is beyond the scope of this chapter to address those serious problems because they require assistance from qualified educational professionals. See Chapter 10 for information about the specialized services parents can pursue for their child to receive in the school setting.

CHILD ACADEMIC SUCCESS PLAN 1: HELPING A CHILD APPRECIATE AND ENJOY READING

YOU HAVE TO READ TO SUCCEED

Eight-year-old Juanita is a typical child in many ways. She goes to school, plays with her friends whenever she can, and enjoys singing in school and church choirs. When it comes to reading, however, Juanita would rather clean her room! Whenever she has "down time" she watches TV or instant messages on the computer. She hates homework and the reading that is involved. Juanita's parents, Maria and Alfonso, are worried about Juanita's lack of interest in reading because they know how important reading is to Juanita's future success.

You may wonder why so much emphasis is put on reading in this book and not on math, writing, social studies, or any other subject? Of course all academic subjects are important, but reading is arguably the most important. To put it bluntly, you need to read to function in life. Simple daily tasks such as understanding traffic signs, following directions on a doctor's prescription, or cooking from a recipe cannot be accomplished if you don't know how to read. Having good reading skills is a very strong predictor of later academic success and employment. Lower reading skill is associated with academic failure, school drop out, under- or unemployment, and even juvenile delinquency. In short, a child has to read to succeed.

Since most parents are not professional teachers, this section will not tell parents how to instruct a child on phonetics or reading comprehension skills. Rather the goal is to suggest ideas on how parents can support their child's reading activity at home. The primary aim is for parents to instill enthusiasm and enjoyment in reading for their child.

Create a "Reading-Friendly" Home Environment

There are many common-sense and practical approaches that a parent can use to create a reading-friendly environment. The following is a list of suggestions that can be used to promote reading in the home:

- Have age- and grade-appropriate books around the house.
- Subscribe to age- and grade-appropriate magazines that are of interest to your child.
- Make sure your child has a comfortable chair to sit in and good lighting for reading.
- Have a bookshelf for your child to collect favorite books and magazines.
- Discuss the value of reading for pleasure and to learn.
- Routinely visit and check out books from the local library.
- Have pencils, markers, papers, and so on available for writing.
- Limit television, video games, and computer time.
- Schedule reading time each day (e.g., 15 minutes for preschoolers, 30–45 minutes for school-age children, and 60 minutes for teens).

Be a Good Reading Model

Children are more likely to read if they see their parents reading. Here are several suggestions on how to be a good reading model:

- Set a good example by reading newspapers, magazines, and books while your child is present.
- Discuss what you are reading with your child.
- Go to the library and check out your own books.

Read Together

One of the best ways to spark enthusiasm for reading in a child is for a parent to read to or with her. Below is a list of good activities and routines to follow in order to promote reading together time:

- Schedule a reading time (e.g., before bed).
- Read age- and grade-level-appropriate books that are of interest to the child.
- Read to your child in an enthusiastic manner.
- Ask your child questions about what is being read.
- Allow your child to point to pictures or text in the book while reading.
- After your child reads or says something about the story, repeat or paraphrase what she said.
- Praise the child for participating in the reading activity.
- Have fun!

LET'S READ SOME MORE

Maria and Alfonso see problems ahead for Juanita if she doesn't learn to appreciate reading instead of dreading it. They decide to make reading a priority for Juanita. To begin with, they make a rule that she can only have 1 hour per day of "screen time," including both TV and computer. They set up a reading corner in Juanita's bedroom with a comfortable chair, good lighting, and a bookshelf for her books. Since Juanita is crazy about horses, her parents subscribe to a horse-related magazine that Juanita said she would like. Juanita is now required to read about 30 minutes per day. Maria and Alfonso also read with her every night before bed for at least 20 minutes, although they often read more because they are having so much fun. One evening, after finishing a book with Alfonso, Juanita actually protested and exclaimed, "Let's read some more!"

CHILD ACADEMIC SUCCESS PLAN 2: TEACHING A CHILD SELF-DIRECTED ACADEMIC BEHAVIOR SKILLS

NOT WORKING UP TO POTENTIAL

Thirteen-year-old Sean does very well on standardized achievement tests, yet receives poor grades at school. Apparently he has the ability and he is learning, but he doesn't do the day-to-day work necessary to get good grades. Sean's parents, Reiko and Kim, get notes from teachers stating that "Sean is frequently off-task," "Sean doesn't complete assignments," "Sean wastes time," and "Sean is not working up to his potential."

Some children struggle academically because of learning disabilities, while others are quite capable, but don't keep up with the work. Academic underachievement can be the end result in either scenario. Teachers will tell you that academic achievement is equal parts ability and performance. The performance aspect pertains to "producing a product" to demonstrate what has been learned. These products include completing worksheets, handing in assignments, writing papers, and doing well on tests. Many struggling children do not produce products at school very well because they do not have needed "self-directed academic behaviors" in their repertoire. These include organizational and homework skills, as well as the capacity for staying on task to complete work. Child Academic Success Plan 2 gives parents ideas on how to improve these essential skills in their child.

Improving Organizational Skills

You can apply a variety of techniques to help your child develop organizational skills. Younger children will need more monitoring and hands-on help to develop these skills than most older children. The skills you teach will need to be adjusted to your child's age. The following is a list of organizational strategies that may be helpful.

Assignment Notebook System

Teach your child to keep track of her assignments on a daily basis. Obtain a calendar or daily planner. Help her develop a system where she routinely writes down assignments and their due dates. Each day she should write down what was discussed in class that day, what is due the next day, and any long-term assignments that will be due in the future, such as a book report. Guide the child to break down long-term assignments into small steps. For example, with a book report the child could write down a plan such as (1) read the book between Thursday and Sunday, (2) create an outline of the book report on Monday, (3) write a draft on Tuesday, (4) edit the draft on Wednesday, and (5) write a final draft on Thursday. Develop a system where she checks off assignments as they are completed.

Time Budgeting

Teach your child to plan how to use her time wisely. Help her develop a system where she writes down all of the work that needs to be done, on either a daily or a weekly basis, and estimates how much time it will take to complete each task. Then she plans on her calendar how much time she will devote to each assignment and when she will do it. For example, when your child sits down for daily homework, she could write down all of her assignments for that day and allocate a certain amount of time for each assignment. For longer assignments, the planning should be done for an extended time basis. For example, if your child needs to write a paper or do a special project, she could plan and write down a schedule of different steps to accomplish over several weeks (e.g., when to go to the library, when she will complete an outline, when to write a draft, and so on).

Organizational Checklists

Your child can develop organizational checklists with your guidance. This involves listing all the smaller steps that comprise a large task or activity. Your child then checks off each step as it is completed. Organizational checklists can be used for getting ready for school in the morning, getting ready to come home from school at the end of the school day, preparing to do homework, or doing math problems. The **Example: Organizational Checklists** (at the end of the chapter) provide additional ideas.

Improving Your Child's Homework Skills

A child can improve homework skills by developing routines. Below are some helpful routines to follow.

Designate a Home Study Area

Set aside a quiet place for your child to study. This place should be free of distraction, have adequate lighting, and be stocked with necessary school-related supplies (e.g., paper, pencils, erasers, etc.). Ideally, your child would also have this particular area decorated with posters or artwork to make it a desirable place to work in.

Designate a Homework Time

Assign a designated time for homework. For example, you might require your child to study between 5 and 6 P.M. Designate a standard amount of time for homework regardless of whether the child has homework or not (e.g., 30–45 minutes for elementary school-age children and 60 minutes for teens). This reduces the child's tendency to rush or "forget" homework. Your child can review or read during homework time when she does not have an assignment to work on.

Teach Homework Organization

Help your child organize homework each day by seeing what needs to be done, planning how it will be done, and determining how much time to spend on each task.

Take Breaks

Some children benefit from taking periodic breaks during homework. It may be unrealistic to expect your child to sit still and stay on task for 1 hour, so this should be taken into account. If your child has particular difficulty in this area, it may be helpful to study for 10 minutes, take a 5-minute break, study for 10 minutes, take a 5-minute break, or some variation of this pattern. Another idea would be to take short breaks in between specific homework tasks as they are completed.

Help Child

Assist or check your child's work, without doing it for her.

Praise Child

Most homework experts agree that a child should not be paid for studying, but it is important to praise your child for her studying effort. Paying her won't promote a desire to learn for the sake of learning. Praise and encouragement will help inspire a desire to learn in your child. It is wise to **praise your child's efforts** as she pursues academic activities. The focus should be on praising your child for putting in a good day's work, completing an assignment, reading a chapter, and so forth. You should focus less on getting good grades and more on working hard. **If your child is reinforced for her effort and works harder, good grades will follow.**

Teaching a Child to Self-Monitor On-Task Behavior

Many children have short attention spans, get off-task, and therefore have a hard time completing their work. These children often benefit from being trained to "self-monitor" their on-task behavior. This section reviews a self-monitoring procedure that you can initiate at home to help your child learn this important skill and thereby improve work productivity. Usually this self-monitoring exercise would be done during homework time, but could also be used for other tasks (such as doing chores). Self-monitoring for on-task behavior is most successful for children over the age of 8. Children under the age of 8 probably need more external monitoring and reminders by their parents to stay on-task because they are less developmentally capable of doing it on their own.

Step 1: Instruct Child about On-Task Behavior

It is necessary for your child to clearly understand what on-task behavior is. Define on-task behavior for her and model this behavior. For example, with homework, you would explain to your child that on-task behavior means looking at one's work, having the pencil touch the paper, writing, calculating, or reading. It may be helpful to demonstrate physically or model these behaviors.

Step 2: Use Self-Monitoring to Improve On-Task Behavior

The **Staying On-Task** chart (at the end of the chapter) can be used to help your child improve on-task behavior. The first step is to designate a task for your child to complete and a time interval during which the task will be completed. For example, your child could self-monitor on-task behavior while completing an hour's worth of homework. Your child is to make an effort to stay on-task while attempting to complete the task. After the time interval has passed, both your child and you rate how well she stayed on task according to the 5-point rating scale described on the Staying On-Task chart.

At first, it is most helpful to focus on whether or not your child's rating matches your rating. If desired, you could give your child a reward if her rating matches your rating. (See the Appendix for more ideas about rewards for children.) In the beginning it is not so important that your child actually improve on-task behavior, but that her ratings match yours, which shows she is becoming a better observer of her own behavior. By focusing on matching, your child will become more aware of when she is on- or off-task. Keep up the matching procedure until your child is good at self-observation of on-task behavior.

The next step is to use the Staying On-Task chart to improve on-task behavior. This would be accomplished by the child actually obtaining ratings of 3, 4, or 5 on the chart. You could provide your child a reward if she achieves a good rating on the Staying On-Task chart. (See the Appendix for more ideas about rewards for children.)

WORKING UP TO POTENTIAL

Back to Sean, Reiko, and Kim: Reiko and Kim decide to help Sean develop skills necessary for academic success. At first, they focus on strengthening his on-task behavior through self-monitoring training. Sean uses the Staying On-Task chart for homework. Reiko helps Sean develop organizational checklists for when he sits down to do homework. Kim makes sure that Sean uses his daily planner to keep track of homework assignments. Gradually, Sean shows success in developing self-directed academic behaviors. Everyone is pleased when Sean's report card shows improved grades.

CHILD ACADEMIC SUCCESS PLAN 3: BEING INVOLVED IN A CHILD'S SCHOOLING

WHAT'S GOING ON?

Eleven-year-old Michelle used to do well in school, but this year her grades have fallen, and she is getting in trouble for goofing off and wasting time. Michelle's parents, Amanda and Kevin, both work full-time in demanding jobs. Trying to manage work and keep up with Michelle and her two younger siblings' schedules is a challenge. Family life is hectic to say the least. Her parents are puzzled as to why Michelle's latest report card was not as good as usual. Today, Ms. Robins, Michelle's teacher, called Amanda at work and told her that Michelle hasn't completed any homework for over two weeks. Amanda was shocked at this news. Later that evening Amanda mentioned to Michelle that the teacher informed her of Michelle's poor homework completion and asked, "What's going on?"

General Tips

One of the strongest predictors of a child's academic success is parental involvement with schooling. This section gives ideas on how parents can get more involved with their child around school-related activities.

Communicate to Your Child That You Value Education

Without lecturing, it is helpful to discuss the value of an education with your child on a routine basis. Perhaps more important, however, is that she sees you actively involved in some sort of a learning process yourself. Your involvement in a learning process could be formal, such as taking classes, or more informal, such as watching educational TV and reading books. It is best if your child sees you practicing what you preach in terms of promoting the value of education.

Maintain Ongoing Contact with School Personnel

Whenever possible, try to attend school functions. This includes school conferences, day visits, meetings, and activities that your child is involved with during and after the school day. Many schools have websites where teachers post notes to parents and provide information about homework assignments. Check the website on a regular basis to keep tabs on what is going on in your child's classroom. To be truly involved, it is a good idea to have active and ongoing contact with school personnel, not just when problems arise.

Assist Your Child with Academic Activities

This means being available to help and support your child regarding homework or planning for school-related activities. You can accomplish this by assisting her in making decisions, planning, and organizing school tasks and activities.

Home–School Note System

It can be very helpful to strengthen the ties between school and home by forming a collaborative relationship between school personnel and parents. When school and home work together, a child is likely to be more successful with academic endeavors.

A home–school note system often can help you monitor your child's progress at school. To implement this procedure, you and your child's teacher agree on a system of ongoing communication between home and school. Many teachers already have systems developed for this purpose.

The basic idea is to have a note passed between parents and teachers each day with your child acting as the delivery agent. Usually a form is developed that targets a specific behavior or behaviors (e.g., stay on-task, complete classroom work, cooperate with teacher) and how well your child did on that behavior each day (e.g., poor, fair, good) The teacher signs the form at the end of the day and sends it home via the child. At first it may be hard for your child to "remember" to bring the note home, but over time she can learn to do the home–school note delivery successfully. In some instances, it is necessary to administer a mild punishment if your child continuously "forgets" the note. You may choose to administer a reward or negative consequence at home, depending on your child's behavior at school that day.

The sample **Home–School Note** (at the end of the chapter) can be modified to meet your child's unique needs. The behaviors targeted on the home–school note will be different for a younger versus an older child/teen. With an older child/teen you may need to develop an hourly schedule and focus on more sophisticated behaviors such as "participate in positive ways during classroom discussion" or "cooperate with students and teacher."

WORKING TOGETHER

Michelle's parents decide they need to get more involved with her schooling. They talk with Michelle to make a plan. Amanda and Kevin communicate their clear expectation that Michelle needs to make her schoolwork a top priority and that getting a good education is very important in their family. They tell her that they are going to monitor her schoolwork closely and have ongoing communication with her teachers. They make sure to check the school website on a regular basis so they know what Michelle's homework assignments are and can keep track of her grades. They also meet with Ms. Robins to develop a home–school note system to monitor Michelle's progress in algebra more closely. Behaviors targeted in the home–school note include staying on-task, completing assignments, and using class time wisely. Finally, they resolve to be more actively involved with Michelle at school in general. They make a point of attending Michelle's band concert and go to several of her soccer games. After several weeks Amanda and Kevin observe that Michelle is making slow but steady improvement in her grades and behavior at school.

CHARTS FOR CHAPTER 6

EXAMPLE: ORGANIZATIONAL CHECKLISTS

**For Getting Ready for School
in the Morning**

____ Get up at 6:30 A.M.

____ Take a shower

____ Get dressed

____ Eat breakfast

____ Get backpack

____ Catch bus

For Homework

____ Get out all books

____ Sharpen pencil

____ Write down all tasks that need
to be done

____ Do homework

____ Check my work

____ Ask for help if needed

**For Preparing to Come Home
from School**

____ Get backpack

____ Pack all needed books

____ Pack homework calendar

____ Ask teacher to sign home–school note

____ Pack home–school note

____ Catch bus

For Math Worksheet

____ Get out worksheet

____ Look at the "sign" for each math problem

____ Do math problem

____ Ask for help if needed

EXAMPLE: STAYING ON-TASK

Name: *Sean*

Date: *Monday*

Directions: Indicate below what task you will be doing (e.g., school work, cleaning up your room, a special project, etc.) and the time period you will be working on the task. After you have completed the task or after the time period is over, rate yourself as to how well you stayed on-task. Next a parent should rate how well you stayed on-task.

Task to be completed and Time Period

1. **I will work on this task during this time:**
   Homework from 5 P.M.–6 P.M.

Child Evaluation

2. **How well did I stay on-task?** (circle one)

1	2	3	(4)	5
Not at all	A little	OK	Pretty good	Great

Parent Evaluation

3. **How well did child stay on-task?** (circle one)

1	2	3	(4)	5
Not at all	A little	OK	Pretty good	Great

Reward

4. **If my rating matches my parent rating, I get this reward:**
   Stay up late Friday night

OR

5. **If my parent rates me as a 3, 4, 5, I get this reward:**
   Stay up late Friday night

STAYING ON-TASK

Name: _____

Date: _____

Directions: Indicate below what task you will be doing (e.g., school work, cleaning up your room, a special project, etc.) and the time period you will be working on the task. After you have completed the task or after the time period is over, rate yourself as to how well you stayed on-task. Next a parent should rate how well you stayed on-task.

Task to be completed and Time Period

1. **I will work on this task during this time:**

Child Evaluation

2. **How well did I stay on-task?** (circle one)

1	2	3	4	5
Not at all	A little	OK	Pretty good	Great

Parent Evaluation

3. **How well did child stay on-task?** (circle one)

1	2	3	4	5
Not at all	A little	OK	Pretty good	Great

Reward

4. **If my rating matches my parent rating, I get this reward:**

OR

5. **If my parent rates me as a 3, 4, 5, I get this reward:**

EXAMPLE: HOME–SCHOOL NOTE

Name: Michelle _____ Date: May 17 _____

Morning

		Circle one	
Obeyed teacher and classroom rules	Poor	(Fair)	Good
Stayed on-task	(Poor)	Fair	Good
Interacted with peers positively	Poor	Fair	(Good)

Comments: Nice job helping Courtney with math sheet _____

Teacher's signature: Mrs. Pearson _____

Afternoon

		Circle one	
Obeyed teacher and classroom rules	Poor	Fair	(Good)
Stayed on-task	Poor	(Fair)	Good
Interacted with peers positively	Poor	Fair	(Good)

Comments: Great job following instructions in gym class _____

Teacher's signature: Mrs. Pearson _____

Today's homework assignments are:

Math worksheet _____

Read chapter 4 in history book _____

_____

_____

HOME–SCHOOL NOTE

Name: _____   Date: _____

Morning

	Circle one		
Obeyed teacher and classroom rules	Poor	Fair	Good
Stayed on-task	Poor	Fair	Good
Interacted with peers positively	Poor	Fair	Good

Comments: _____

Teacher's signature: _____

Afternoon

	Circle one		
Obeyed teacher and classroom rules	Poor	Fair	Good
Stayed on-task	Poor	Fair	Good
Interacted with peers positively	Poor	Fair	Good

Comments: _____

Teacher's signature: _____

Today's homework assignments are:

_____

_____

_____

_____

Chapter 7

Improving Parent Well-Being

If a parent is stressed out or having personal problems, it is difficult to follow through with all the responsibility and hard work of parenting. Stress for parents often takes the form of personal stress, marital/relationship stress, parenting stress, and lack of social support. **Personal stress** occurs when a parent feels very overwhelmed with life. At its extreme a stressed-out parent may suffer from depression or anxiety and sometimes turn to alcohol or drugs to deal with personal problems. **Marital/relationship stress** is observed when a parent experiences continual conflict with an intimate partner. These problems range from arguments to violence between partners. **Parenting stress** has to do with the ongoing hassles of raising children, which are especially acute when parenting a struggling child. Parents can become burned out from their child's problems. If a parent is experiencing **lack of social support,** he or she feels very alone and has little or no assistance in the day-to-day burdens of parenting. It is especially stressful to be isolated when parenting a struggling child. Too often these forms of stress are also associated with **unhelpful thinking** in parents, such as negative beliefs and assumptions about their child, self, or others.

Different forms of parent stress, as defined above, are serious problems that have the potential to build and escalate. Obviously, increased parent stress coupled with unhelpful thoughts can interfere with parenting. When stressed out, a parent can be ineffective in discipline, and sometimes a strain develops in the parent–child relationship. This disruption in parenting can lead to the increase of behavior and adjustment problems in a child, which in turn is stressful for the parent. The relationship among parent stress, parent

145

thoughts, parenting, and child behavior and adjustment problems is depicted in Figure 7.1. The main lesson from this is that **parents must take steps to reduce their stress and change the way they think in order to be good parents.**

This chapter will provide three Parent Well-Being Success Plans for parents to improve their self-care skills including:

Parent Well-Being Success Plan 1: Improving Parent Stress Management Skills—gives parents common-sense ideas on how to cope better with everyday stresses and personal problems (see pages 147–151).

Parent Well-Being Success Plan 2: Staying Calm with a Stressful Child—has suggestions for staying cool when dealing with challenging child behavior (see pages 151–152).

Parent Well-Being Success Plan 3: Changing Unhelpful Parent Thoughts—assists parents in recognizing, understanding, and changing negative or unhelpful thoughts (see pages 152–154).

These Parent Well-Being Success Plans are a good place to start when a parent is dealing with mild to moderate stress and are applicable in the families of children of all ages. Occasionally a parent may feel under so much

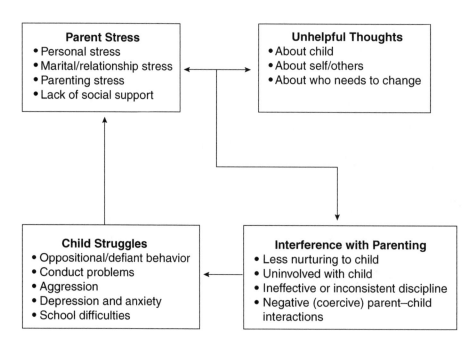

FIGURE 7.1. Parent stress cycle.

stress that self-care strategies may not be enough. **If you are experiencing high stress, it may be helpful to consult a mental health and/or chemical health professional.** If the professional recommends a specific course of treatment, then it would be wise to pursue it. In many instances, individual therapy, chemical dependency treatment, couple or family therapy, and/or medications may be indicated.

PARENT WELL-BEING SUCCESS PLAN 1: IMPROVING PARENT STRESS MANAGEMENT SKILLS

PARENTS UNDER STRESS

John and Judy have been married 12 years. They have two children, 10-year-old Jacob and 8-year-old Sarah. Jacob is a handful who has significant behavior problems at home, at school, and in interacting with his friends in the neighborhood. He is especially defiant at home. He refuses even the smallest requests by his parents. Jacob also starts many fights with his sister. They have resolved that they are going to try to be more consistent and "not let him get his way anymore."

John and Judy have a very busy and hurried lifestyle. To make ends meet, John works a full- and a part-time job. Judy also works full-time and is responsible for most of the household chores. When John is at home, he watches TV and doesn't spend much time with the family. When he does interact, he is grumpy and complains a lot. Judy thinks that John is lazy, and she feels like a single parent because he is so uninvolved in family matters. John and Judy find themselves arguing frequently. Judy has even thought of divorcing John, but has not done so because of the children.

Last Tuesday, after dinner, Judy asked Jacob to clean the dishes off the table and bring them to the sink. By the time Judy made the request, Jacob, Sarah, and John were already watching TV. Judy nagged Jacob several times. She asked John for assistance, but he didn't budge. Finally, after several attempts to get Jacob to clean off the table without any assistance from John, Judy cleaned the table off herself.

The point has already been made that you cannot provide what your child needs unless you manage your own stress and personal problems. Clearly, you need to take care of yourself in order to be available to meet the needs of your child. Below is a discussion of possible ways in which a parent might enhance his or her ability to manage stress.

Stress Management Strategies

What follows are common-sense approaches to manage stress. For the most part these methods can be learned through a self-help format such as this book. Sometimes it is helpful to obtain the assistance of a mental health professional to develop these skills.

Relax

Learn to relax your body through various relaxation procedures. It may be helpful to consult professional publications and/or a mental health professional to learn specific relaxation strategies.

Take Time Away from Family Responsibility

It can be rejuvenating to schedule time for you to pursue an activity or interest. You may need to arrange for a babysitter, or, if there are two parents, you might want to take turns caring for your children so that each parent can get out occasionally.

Take Time to Be with Spouse/Partner (If Applicable)

If parents spend enjoyable time with each other without their children around, they may improve their relationship. It does not have to cost money and may be as simple as a walk or drive together. Brainstorm with your spouse/partner about enjoyable things to do together and make the time to do them.

Spend Special Time with Child

Parents and children these days are so busy they find it hard to have quality time together. Make an effort to spend time with your child to build a quality relationship. You will have fewer problems getting along if you schedule special time. See Chapter 8 for ideas to promote involvement with your child.

Seek Out Social Support

Parents who are feeling overwhelmed and isolated can benefit from seeking out active support from family members, neighbors, or mental health professionals. This support could involve getting babysitters, talking and sharing feelings with friends or family members, asking for help from friends or family members, or even participating in individual therapy.

Schedule Pleasant Events

Stress can be relieved by scheduling specific pleasant events. For example, you may want to attend a concert, go out to dinner with a friend, take the dog for a walk with your children, or attend a baseball game with your son or daughter.

Develop Good Health Habits

It is universally accepted that increasing one's exercise level, eating a healthy diet, getting enough rest, and relaxing periodically can improve one's ability to cope with stress. Consult professional publications and/or a physician regarding a health promotion program for you.

Use Effective Problem Solving

If you find yourself continually dealing with the same problems, then utilizing problem-solving strategies could be helpful. In Chapters 4 and 8 information is reviewed regarding problem-solving skills for the child and family. Review of those chapters may give you ideas about developing your own problem-solving skills.

Think Accurately and Rationally

Often our stress is caused by the way we think about ourselves, others, and the events of life. You can learn to reevaluate and change unhelpful thoughts. We will be focusing on changing thoughts related to one's child and parenting abilities in the last section of this chapter. Again, you might consider consulting professional publications and/or a mental health professional to learn about how to think more accurately and rationally.

Learn to Control Anger

Parents often get very angry at their child or spouse/partner when dealing with struggling children. A parent learning to control anger can be helpful. Chapter 3 describes anger management for children, and in the next section of this chapter we review staying calm with stressful children. Some of these ideas can help a parent manage anger too. However, if you have a big anger problem, you should consult a mental health professional.

Join a Parent Support Group

I have been conducting parent groups for many years. These groups focus on skills training but also allow parents to share "war stories" and obtain support from each other. Many parents comment that the support and opportunity to share experiences are very beneficial (sometimes more beneficial than the skills training!). If you have a child with serious, chronic behavior and/or adjustment problems, you may benefit from joining a parent support group. Consult with a local mental health professional or social service agency about such groups in your community.

Plan Lifestyle Changes

The above examples of stress management really are about changing one's lifestyle. Changing a lifestyle involves much effort and planning to make it work. It may be helpful for the parents to sit down together each Sunday and plan the following week by scheduling stress management activities and priorities. For example, the parents could schedule times for going out on "dates" with each other, a mother might schedule visiting her sister on Thursday evening, or a father might arrange which weekday mornings he will exercise.

LET'S TAKE CARE OF OURSELVES

Back to John and Judy: John and Judy have become familiarized with parent stress management ideas through a parent support group they have been attending. One day they sit down to discuss how they might be able to manage their stress better. They decide that at least twice a month they are going to try to go out for dinner, a movie, or some other enjoyable activity. John will schedule and arrange babysitters for these two monthly rendezvous. John also has decided that he will consult a mental health professional for an evaluation because he realizes he is not as happy as he would like to be. Both parents decide that they will take turns every other morning exercising while the other takes charge of the responsibilities of breakfast, getting the children ready for school, and so forth. Judy has decided that she will try to go out with her sister once a month because she finds her sister to be very supportive and a lot of fun. John and Judy are also trying to use techniques to stay calm when dealing with Jacob and the parenting challenges he presents. In the future, they hope that their stress management techniques will help them feel more capable of disciplining Jacob and helping him learn to be more cooperative.

PARENT WELL-BEING SUCCESS PLAN 2: STAYING CALM WITH A STRESSFUL CHILD

I'VE HAD ENOUGH OUT OF YOU!

Priscilla and Randy are the proud parents of 11-year-old Lori. Lori is so difficult at home that her parents frequently find themselves quite angry with her. Everything is a battle with Lori, from eating her breakfast in the morning to going to bed at night. Lori mostly dawdles, but increasingly she just refuses to do what her parents tell her to. Last night Randy told Lori to turn off the TV and get ready for bed. She said "uh huh," but just sat there. After a minute, Randy was boiling mad. He shouted "I've had enough out of you!" He pulled Lori by the arm to her room, causing Lori to cry and Priscilla to come running to see what was the matter.

Because the major focus of this book is about parenting challenging children, it is important to address the stress of interacting with them. Parents often find themselves angry at or overwhelmed by their child. Learning techniques for staying calm with a difficult child on a day-to-day basis may be helpful. **Staying calm while interacting with your challenging child involves being aware of and controlling how you react to stressful events with your child.**

Try to be more aware of your body, thoughts, and actions while interacting with your child. For example, imagine you are getting ready to go to a dentist appointment and you need to get out of the house soon, but your child is leisurely getting ready to go. You might feel tense, your heart rate goes up, and you breathe rapidly. Your thoughts might be unhelpful (e.g., "That brat!" or "Why do we have to go through this same old stuff everyday?" or "I'm going to ground him for a year this time!"). In this scenario it would not be too surprising if you end up yelling at and threatening your child out of frustration. The **Staying Calm** chart (at the end of the chapter) displays typical body, thought, and action responses that occur when dealing with a stressful child. Make a list of typical stressful events that regularly occur with your child and how you usually react as far as your body, thoughts, and actions are concerned.

Staying calm involves learning to control your body, thoughts, and actions in the face of parenting stress. This means learning to relax your body, think helpful thoughts, and take effective action when under stress from your child. The Staying Calm chart summarizes techniques you can use to control your body, thoughts, and actions when dealing with stressful situations involving your child. You could post this chart in your house to remind you what to do. It's also a good idea to let your child know that you are working on staying calm because then you are being a good role model on how to handle stress. More information about anger management, which is very similar to staying calm with stressful children, can be found in Chapter 3.

CHILL OUT

After a big fight with Lori, Priscilla and Randy sit down to discuss what they can do about her behavior. They realize that first they need to handle their own frustration better with Lori so they can then be more effective in handling her behavior. They decide to follow the suggestions found in the Staying Calm chart. They agree that when they observe each other getting too mad with Lori, they can cue each other to "chill out." With that cue, they know to apply the strategies in the chart. The parents use this procedure for several weeks and note that they are less and less upset with Lori.

PARENT WELL-BEING SUCCESS PLAN 3: CHANGING UNHELPFUL PARENT THOUGHTS

I GIVE UP

James and Shayla are the parents of 16-year-old Tanya. Ever since kindergarten they have been getting notes and calls from teachers about Tanya's disruptive behavior in the classroom. At home, she has been a significant challenge since day one. She has seen psychologists and psychiatrists and has been involved in special education services at school. Recently, Tanya has been hanging out with her friends and is hardly ever at home. She doesn't tell her parents where she is going, what she will be doing, or who she is with. Her parents wonder if she's starting to experiment with marijuana.

One Saturday night, after Tanya missed yet another midnight curfew, James and Shayla were having a conversation. They were both very frustrated. Shayla said, "I have failed as a parent," and "There's no hope for Tanya." James responded, "Shayla is such a brat," and "I give up!"

Research and clinical experience shows that **parent thoughts affect parent–child relationships and are indirectly related to the child's development of**

behavioral and adjustment problems. Some parents think their child is the cause of the family's problems. Other parents may expect their child to do things that are too advanced for his capabilities. There are parents who believe their child's behavior is out of their control and that there is nothing they can do. Parents can blame themselves, their spouse/partner, or school personnel for their child's struggles.

Whether or not there is some truth to these thoughts, they are not constructive and can lead to additional child and family problems. You've heard the saying "you are what you eat." Well it's also true that "you are what you think." Your thoughts about your child, self, and others relate to how you behave in a parenting situation. For these reasons, it is very important that parents examine and, if needed, change their thoughts.

A parent can change the way he or she thinks. This next section helps parents identify and understand the significance of unhelpful thoughts and change them to more helpful thoughts.

Step 1: Identify and Understand Unhelpful Thoughts

The first step is identifying one's own unhelpful thoughts. Do a self-evaluation of your thoughts by completing the **Unhelpful Parent Thoughts** chart (at the end of the chapter). The next step is to understand the unhelpful nature of these thoughts. This can be accomplished by asking yourself the questions found at the bottom of the chart.

As an example, let's examine the thought "My child acts up on purpose," using the questions from the bottom of the chart. **What is unhelpful about this thought?** There may be times when your child misbehaves without even being aware of it. Your own parenting behavior may also be contributing to the child's misbehavior. If you have this thought, you may not be examining your own contribution to the problem. Even if it is true, is it helpful to keep thinking the thought? **How would this thought influence my behavior toward my child?** If you assume your child misbehaves on purpose, you are more likely to blame him, get angry with him, or punish him. **How would my behavior affect my child?** If you think of your child as misbehaving on purpose, it could lead you to blame or punish, and it sends a negative message to him. He is more likely to blame himself, and your behavior may tell the child that he is not good enough. Over time, your behavior could possibly lower your child's self-esteem. Ask yourself similar questions for other unhelpful thoughts that you have checked off for yourself.

Step 2: Counter with Helpful Thoughts

Once you understand the unhelpful nature of these thoughts, you can make changes. A technique known as "countering" is often useful in this regard. **Countering involves rethinking your thoughts in a more helpful manner.** To accomplish this, you can use the **Helpful Parent Thoughts** chart (at the end of the chapter). The counter thoughts listed on the Helpful chart correspond directly to the unhelpful thoughts on the Unhelpful chart. For example, the previously listed Unhelpful Thought 1 can be countered with Helpful Thought 1.

Carefully examine the helpful counter thoughts. Ask yourself the questions at the bottom of the Helpful Parent Thoughts chart. Chances are your answers to the questions pertaining to helpful thoughts are more favorable than your answers regarding the unhelpful thoughts.

LET'S GIVE IT OUR BEST SHOT

Back to James, Shayla, and Tanya: At one point, James remembers that he has read about parent thoughts with challenging children. He realizes that his thoughts are not very helpful and states, "You know, honey, we can't just give up. This is our daughter we're talking about. We need to keep trying." During a long discussion, James and Shayla realize they can't predict the future but that if they don't try something, their fears may come true. They realize that it doesn't help to blame themselves. Rather they need to take some action. At that point, James and Shayla start thinking about different ways in which they might approach the challenge of parenting Tanya.

CHARTS FOR CHAPTER 7

STAYING CALM

1. **Recognize Stress**—Be aware of stress "signals."

   Body signals
   - Breathing/heart rate increased
   - Tense muscles
   - Increased sweating
   - Face turns red
   - Body feels hot

   Thought signals
   - "That brat!"
   - "I'm not going to take any more!"
   - "I'm a worthless parent."
   - "I can't handle this!"
   - "I hate him/her."
   - "I give up."

   Action signals
   - Punch/hit
   - Yell/threaten
   - Cry
   - Tremble
   - Withdraw

2. **Relax Your Body**—Do deep breathing, tense and release muscles, count to 10, and so forth.

3. **Use "Coping Self-Talk"**—Examples of coping self-talk include the following:

   - "Take it easy."
   - "Don't let it bug you."
   - "I can handle this."
   - "I'm going to be OK."
   - "Stay cool."
   - "Relax."
   - "I'll try my best."

4. **Taking Effective Action**—Walk away, ignore it, take a walk, try to discuss it, express feelings, think of new ways to solve the problem.

UNHELPFUL PARENT THOUGHTS

Listed below are a variety of common thoughts that parents of struggling children may have. Read each thought and indicate how frequently that thought (or a similar thought) typically occurs for you over an average week. There are no right or wrong answers to these questions. Use the 3-point rating scale to help you answer these questions.

1	2	3
Rarely	**Sometimes**	**Often**

Unhelpful Thoughts about the Child

1. ____ My child is behaving like a brat.
2. ____ My child acts up on purpose.
3. ____ My child is the cause of most of our family problems.
4. ____ My child's future is bleak.
5. ____ My child should behave like other children. I shouldn't have to make allowances for my child.

Unhelpful Thoughts about Self/Others

6. ____ It is my fault that my child has a problem.
7. ____ It is his/her fault (other parent) that my child is this way.
8. ____ I can't make mistakes in parenting my child.
9. ____ I give up. There is nothing more I can do for my child.
10. ____ I have no control over my child. I have tried everything.

Unhelpful Thoughts about Who Needs to Change

11. ____ My child is the one who needs to change. All of us would be better off if my child would change.
12. ____ I am the one who needs to change. My family would be better off if I would change.
13. ____ My spouse/partner needs to change. We would all be better off if he/she would change.
14. ____ The teacher needs to change. We would be better off if he/she would change.
15. ____ Medications are the answer. Medications will change my child.

For each thought you rated a 3, ask yourself the following questions:

1. ____ What is unhelpful about this thought?
2. ____ How would this thought influence my behavior toward my child?
3. ____ How would my behavior affect my child?

HELPFUL PARENT THOUGHTS

Listed below are "counter" thoughts that parents can think instead of unhelpful thoughts. Unhelpful Thought #1 corresponds to Helpful Thought #1 and so on. Compare the unhelpful thoughts to the helpful thoughts.

Helpful Thoughts about the Child

1. ____ My child is behaving positively too.

2. ____ It doesn't matter whose fault it is. What matters are solutions to problems.

3. ____ It is not just my child. I also play a role in the problem.

4. ____ I'm being irrational. I have no proof that my child will continue to have problems. I need to wait for the future.

5. ____ I can't just expect my child to behave. My child needs to be taught how to behave.

Helpful Thoughts about Self/Others

6. ____ It doesn't help to blame myself. I will focus on solutions to the problem.

7. ____ It doesn't matter whose fault it is. I will focus on solutions to the problems.

8. ____ My child is perhaps more challenging to parent than others, and therefore I will make mistakes. I need to accept the fact that I am going to make mistakes.

9. ____ I have to parent my child. I have no choice. I need to think of new ways to parent my child.

10. ____ My belief that I have no control over my child might be contributing to the problem. Many things are in my control. I need to figure out what I can do to parent my child.

Helpful Thoughts about Who Needs to Change

11. ____ My child is not the only one who needs to change. We all need to change.

12. ____ I am not the only one who needs to change. We all need to change.

13. ____ My spouse/partner is not the only one who needs to change. We all need to change.

14. ____ The teacher is not the only one who needs to change. We all need to work together.

15. ____ Medications may help, but will not solve the problems. We will also need to work hard to cope with the problems.

Ask yourself the following questions about these helpful thoughts:

1. ____ What is helpful about this thought?

2. ____ How would this thought influence my behavior toward my child?

3. ____ How would my behavior affect my child?

Chapter 8

Improving Family Relationships

Perhaps nothing is more important to a child's development than having strong relationships with parents and a supportive family. Research reveals that parent–child relationship strains and family difficulties are associated with a struggling child's problems, while close parent–child bonds and constructive family interactions predict the development of a successful child. Of course the family will be strengthened as a natural byproduct of carrying out the skills training previously described in this book. It can also help, however, to focus directly on building and strengthening parent–child and family relationships as discussed in this chapter.

Three Family Relationship Success Plans for boosting the parent–child bond and family interactions are presented in this chapter:

Family Relationship Success Plan 1: Improving the Parent–Child Bond— offers ideas to increase positive feelings between parent and child and for paying attention to positive child behavior (see pages 162–167).

Family Relationship Success Plan 2: Improving Family Interactions— presents methods to strengthen important family skills such as communication, problem solving, and conflict resolution (see pages 168–174).

Family Relationship Success Plan 3: Developing Family Routines and Rituals— suggests ways that a family can make daily family life more organized and meaningful (see pages 175–177).

Although the three Family Relationship Success Plans are important for all families, one plan or the other may be better suited for families with different age children. Family Relationship Success Plan 1, improving the parent–child relationship, is fine for families with a younger or school-age child but can also be useful with families of an older child or teen where the parent–child relationship has deteriorated. The skills training methods pertaining to positive family interactions in Family Relationship Success Plan 2 require more participation from the child and focus on family skills that are increasingly important as a child grows older. Therefore, Family Relationship Success Plan 2 will be most helpful for a family with an older child or teen. Family Relationship Success Plan 3 pertains to making ongoing family life more organized and predictable, as well as building a sense of family, and is applicable to families with young children and/or teens.

FAMILY RELATIONSHIP SUCCESS PLAN 1: IMPROVING THE PARENT–CHILD BOND

GROWING APART

Marcia is a busy single mother who works many hours per week in her own restaurant business. She has an 8-year-old son, Carlos, with ADHD. Marcia's life feels overwhelming. There is way too much to do—work, housekeeping, errands, and so on. Occasionally Marcia needs a break and relaxes by reading or going out with a friend. There doesn't seem to be enough time for Carlos. He does a lot of independent things around the house like playing, drawing, and reading, yet Marcia often doesn't pay much attention to him because she has so much work to do. Sometimes she'll ask Carlos to do household chores such as clean his room or clear the dishes. Carlos seems to drag his feet and rarely completes requested tasks unless Marcia nags him. Marcia and Carlos frequently argue and get into power struggles about household chores. Marcia thinks Carlos is too argumentative, which leads her to avoid spending time with him. Marcia is concerned that she and Carlos are growing apart.

Child and family experts universally agree that parents who are involved with their child and attend to her positive behavior are more likely to have a successful child. The ideas below enable a parent to make a purposeful effort to be involved with their child, and contingently give her positive attention for "good" behavior.

Positive Activity Scheduling

Positive activity scheduling can be used to increase involvement and to improve positive parent–child interactions. It requires a parent to **incorporate child-directed activities into the average week.** Child-directed activities are the child's idea, and the parent lets the child be in charge of how the activity unfolds. For example, a young child may choose to play in the sandbox with trucks, while an older child/teen may choose to play catch or make cookies. During child-directed activities, the parent behaves in a manner that builds a relationship with a child (described below).

Positive activity scheduling is accomplished through a four-step procedure:

Step 1: List Activities

List as many activities as possible that your child enjoys doing with you that can be accomplished in 30 minutes or less. Let your child have the most input into the activities to make sure they are very appealing to her.

Examples of activities that work well are:

- Go for a walk
- Ride bikes
- Play a game
- Play with cars/dolls
- Play catch
- Play one-on-one basketball
- Talk
- Go for a drive
- Bowl
- Spontaneous activity
- Build something
- Bake/cook something

Step 2: Schedule "Appointments" with Child

Schedule two or more 30-minute appointments per week when you and your child will engage in one or more of the above activities together (indicate day, date, and time). It works best if you and your child agree on a time and mark it on a calendar. If something comes up and you can't keep the appointment, be sure to reschedule it.

Step 3: Emphasize Relationship Building Parent Behavior

During the activity, **allow your child to direct or be in charge of the play or activity.**

While your child is leading the play or activity, **try to increase praising, describing, and touching parent behaviors as follows:**

Praising—verbally reinforcing the child during the activity.
- "That looks good."
- "You did a nice job."
- "Way to go."
- "Good idea."
- "That's great!"
- "It looks nice."

Describing—comments that describe what the child is doing, how she might be feeling, what she is experiencing, or where she is during the activity.
- "You're looking at the toys."
- "You caught the ball!"
- "You look happy!"
- "You're hiding."
- "You seem to be mad."
- "It looks like you're thinking."

Touching—any positive physical contact with the child during the activity.
- Hugs
- Kisses
- Touching on the shoulder
- Patting the head

While your child is leading the play or activity, **reduce or avoid questions, commands, and criticism as follows:**

Questions—asking the child what she is doing, why she is doing it, and so forth during the activity.
- "Why did you throw the ball?"
- "How about if we play a game?"
- "Why are you looking so mad?"

Commands—telling the child what to do during the activity.
- "Put the dolls in the house."
- "Shake the dice."

- "You bat and I'll pitch."
- "Take a walk with me."

Criticisms—criticizing the child's behavior during the activity.

- "That doesn't look right."
- "I'll show you how to do it right."
- "Try harder next time."
- "You're supposed to do it this way."

Try interacting with your child in the manner described above. You'll notice that she appreciates and responds to the positive parenting behaviors and may become upset, or at least somewhat tense, when you are engaging in the negative parenting behaviors. This is not to say that parents should never ask questions, give commands, or criticize their child. These parent behaviors, however, are not necessary or helpful during child-directed positive activity times.

Step 4: Evaluate Effects of Activity

After the activity has been completed, it is helpful for you and your child to discuss your observations and feelings about the time you spent together. Listen actively to what your child has to say and offer as much positive feedback to your child as possible.

Try this for several weeks to "get things going." After that, it may be automatic for you and your child to interact in this positive way during play and special time activities.

Special Talk Time

Every child can benefit from having a parent who really listens to her. The purpose of Special Talk Time is to talk with the child about what she is experiencing and going through. During these special conversation times, **the goal is to focus completely on your child and strive to understand how she is feeling.** It is okay to ask your child some questions, but primarily strive to create an atmosphere in which she feels free to talk to you about whatever is on her mind. Try to get your child to talk about what she is doing, what her interests are, and how she feels about problems that she may be experiencing and successes she may have had recently.

It may be helpful to schedule Special Talk Time with your child to make sure that these conversation times actually happen. One good idea is to get into a routine of asking your child these things each day at dinner or just before bed.

With busy teens, it is especially hard to set aside time to talk. The alert parent will recognize when opportunities for dialogue emerge and take advantage of them. This might include talking in the car, while shopping, or when doing chores around the house together.

Be Available and Do Special Activities

To be truly involved, you must demonstrate that you are there for your child. If you are involved, your child will seek you out when really needed. **It's important to make a great effort to be involved in your child's activities and interests.** Try to attend teacher conferences, watch athletic games, attend dance recitals, go to band concerts, or attend any other activity your child may participate in. By doing so, you are demonstrating that you care for and are involved with your child.

It can also be helpful occasionally to schedule alone time to help build a special relationship. Spending a large block of time one-on-one with your child can sometimes accomplish this objective. Examples of these activities are going out to dinner, a weekend camping trip, or a brief vacation. These activities provide opportunities to build and strengthen parent–child relationships.

Parent Involvement at School

The research is quite clear in showing that a child is more likely to succeed in school if her parents are involved in her schooling. See Chapter 6 for suggestions on how parents can get more involved as it relates to their child's education and school experiences. A byproduct of these efforts is that the parent–child bond will be enhanced when a parent gets involved with school.

Noticing Good Behavior

Parents often do not notice when their child is behaving positively. It is a fact that noticing positive child behavior not only can increase the child's positive behavior, but can also improve the parent–child relationship. A fairly simple procedure can be used by a parent to notice a child's positive behavior and to make sure the child knows that she is being noticed.

A "Good Behavior Box" can be a helpful way to acknowledge a child's positive behavior. Keep a box on a counter, refrigerator, table, or other convenient place in your home and label it the Good Behavior Box. When you notice your child behaving positively (e.g., sharing, sitting quietly, or helping with a household chore), take out a piece of paper, write a brief note of what you saw, and put the note in the box. It is a good idea to tell your child that you are putting the note in the box. At the end of the day, spend time with your child reviewing all the notes in the box. Make sure your child understands that you have noticed her positive behavior; in so doing, she will also become more aware of that behavior.

Two-to-One Rule for Parent Comments

Researchers have gone into homes and observed daily parent–child interactions. They found that on an average day a parent makes many comments and gives many directions to a child. On some days a parent might give literally hundreds of comments and directions to the child! This ongoing commentary provides ample opportunity for a parent either to create distance or to improve closeness between parent and child and to shape the child's behavior. If the commentary is mostly negative (e.g., "Stop that." "Why do you have to do that?" "There you go again." "How many times must I tell you?"), then a wall between parent and child can build up. If the commentary is mostly positive (e.g., "Good job." "I like the fact you tried to do your best." "You are smart." "I like when you help out."), then good feelings develop between parent and child.

Of course a child will need to be told to do some things and will need reprimanding, but a focus on the positive is needed. **It is recommended that you make a purposeful effort to make twice as many positive comments as negative comments to your child.** This two-to-one rule for parent comments is designed to improve positive feelings between a parent and child and can go a long way toward shaping desirable behavior in the child.

GROWING CLOSER

Back to Marcia and Carlos: Marcia decides to take some action to turn things around. She sets aside several times each week for "special time" with Carlos. She targets Carlos's independent play activity as something she should praise and notice and uses a Good Behavior Box to accomplish this. She is also going to try to get more involved in his school and sports activities. After Marcia and Carlos are feeling better about one another, she intends to implement some different discipline techniques as well.

FAMILY RELATIONSHIP SUCCESS PLAN 2: IMPROVING FAMILY INTERACTIONS

I'M SICK OF YOU

Steve and Martha are the parents of 14-year-old Mike. It's a Friday night, and Mike is about to go out for the evening. The following discussion takes place in the family kitchen just before he leaves:

MIKE: I am going to Jeff's house for his birthday party.

STEVE: OK. Be home by 11 o'clock.

MIKE: (*annoyed and voice raised*) You've got to be kidding me! It's Friday and it's Jeff's birthday. I'm not coming in at 11:00. Jeff said his parents will let everyone stay until 1 A.M. Why can't I?

MARTHA: (*angry and firm tone*) We've told you time and time again that you need to be in by 11 o'clock on weekends. Why do we have to have this argument over and over? If you don't get in by 11 o'clock, then you're not going to get to bed on time, you'll stay up too late, and you won't get enough sleep. When I was your age, I had to be in much earlier than you do. You have a lot more privileges than I did too. If my father set a curfew, I obeyed it. You're starting a pattern here that's . . .

MIKE: (*interrupting with an arguing tone*) Mom, I don't care what you did. There is no reason why I can't stay out until 1:00 like everyone else.

STEVE: (*to Mike, voice raised*) I'm sick of you and all of your arguing. You cause so many problems in this house.

MIKE: (*angry*) I'm sick of you too. You guys are so damn unfair!

MARTHA: This is just another example of you thinking you can run the show. You'd better shape up, young man!

It is no surprise that stressed-out families often have members who interact negatively with one another. Families with poor communication skills often find themselves blaming, putting each other down, not listening, and so forth. Families that are poor problem solvers find themselves repeatedly trying to solve the same problems over and over using ineffective means. Many stressed-out families also find it difficult to resolve conflict with each other. They tend to escalate each other's angry behavior and sometimes find themselves yelling or even getting into physical fights. Families characterized by these types of interactions are more likely to have a struggling child or teen.

Teach Family Communication Skills

Many families in distress tend to be vague, blame each other, talk on and on, interrupt each other, put each other down, yell, or get off the topic. **Good communication skills are necessary to be able to solve family problems and resolve family conflicts.**

Step 1: Introduce Family Communication Skills to Family

To introduce the idea of improving communication skills to the family, it is necessary to have a meeting with all family members. This meeting should be at a convenient time for everyone. It is absolutely necessary that there be no particular problem discussed and that everyone feels good about being with each other. Don't introduce these skills and try to resolve a big problem at the same time.

Give each member of the family a copy of the **Family Communication Skills** chart (at the end of the chapter). Everyone should look over the chart carefully. First, discuss the "DON'Ts." Ask each family member to do self-evaluation to determine which DON'Ts apply to him or her. As long as the tone of the meeting remains positive, family members can give each other feedback about specific DON'Ts they see in each other. The next step is for each family member to declare one or two "DOs" that they will work on while trying to improve communication within the family. Usually, the DOs selected to work on are the opposite of the DON'Ts each member views as a problem for him or her. The Family Communication Skills chart is designed with the DON'Ts opposite the corresponding DOs.

Step 2: Practice Family Communication Skills

It is helpful if family members take turns demonstrating and role playing examples of the DON'Ts and the DOs. For example, you may role play a "lecture" or "sermon" such as "It is important for you to clean up your room when I tell you. If you don't start learning how to clean up now, you will probably be a slob for the rest of your life. You will never be able to get a good job, get married, or have a family if you don't know how to clean up after yourself. When I was your age, my parents always made me clean up, and I did not give them any trouble . . . " Next, try to model a brief and direct approach to the same problem by saying, "I want you to clean up your room right now." A child might demonstrate poor listening such as sitting back in his chair, crossing his arms, and staring away. He could then show better listening such as leaning forward, giving feedback, and making good eye contact. Ideally the family members would take turns practicing the DON'Ts and the corresponding DOs in a similar manner. Encourage family members to coach one another as they practice specific skills.

At first, practice should be somewhat formal and done with neutral or easy problems and situations. The family could conduct another meeting or use the communication skills spontaneously to solve an easy problem. It will be helpful if all family members have the Family Communication Skills chart in their hands as they try to discuss something. Examples of neutral or easy problems to discuss would be what to watch on TV that night or planning how each family member will get to a sibling's playoff baseball game that evening. Practice the communication skills and give each other feedback about DON'Ts and DOs. Practice the skills until family members feel they have learned them.

One exercise a family could try is to audio- or videotape a family discussion. While taping, practice using the communication skills discussing an easy topic. Play back the recording to review and learn how to improve family communication further.

Step 3: Use Family Communication Skills in Real Life

After the family has practiced and learned the communication skills, the family could try to use them to solve real-life problems. It would be helpful, again, if the family members had the Family Communications Skills chart in their hands while carrying on the discussion. Examples of real problems to discuss would be homework, rules of the house, curfew, parents' concerns regarding a child's grades, and a child's concerns regarding parents' rules.

Several strategies can be employed to make sure family members learn and use communication skills. One idea is to post copies of the Family Communication Skills chart in conveniently accessible places within the home. For example, posting the chart on a refrigerator or a bulletin board might be helpful. Another idea is to review and discuss the communication skills periodically to maintain them because many family members use communication skills for a while but later forget them.

Teach Family Problem-Solving Skills

A sure sign a family is having problems is when members can't solve day-to-day problems. Families who are having difficulties seem to hash over the same problems repeatedly. The goal of family problem solving is to help families define problems and then actually use the solution effectively. **A family is advised to develop good family communication skills (see preceding section) before trying family problem solving.**

Step 1: Introduce Family Problem-Solving Skills to Family

As with family communication skills training, the first step is to conduct a family meeting that is convenient for everyone and where everyone is feeling good about being together.

Next give everyone a copy of the **Family Problem Solving** chart (at the end of the chapter). Family members should discuss how good they think their family currently is in solving family problems. Family members should determine whether or not they want to work toward a goal of improving family problem solving. Then review all the steps and make sure that everyone understands them.

Step 2: Practice Family Problem-Solving Skills

After the family problem-solving skills have been introduced, it is a good idea for family members to practice using them to solve neutral or easy problems. At first, try to solve a fun, contrived problem such as how to spend $10,000 that your family just won in the lottery. Next try to solve a real-life, easy problem such as deciding what to have for dinner, where to go for an evening outing, or what show to watch on TV.

As with family communication skills, it may be helpful to make an audio- or videotape of a family problem-solving episode. The family could review the recording to give each other constructive feedback and to learn.

Step 3: Use Family Problem Solving in Real Life

The final step is to use family problem solving with real-life problems. It may be helpful to have the Family Problem Solving chart available to family members while discussing these difficult issues. It is critical that family members go through each step very carefully, one at a time. It is also essential that family members use good communication skills while trying to solve these problems.

One note of caution about family problem solving: **Make sure your child understands that all disputes are not open to negotiation.** The parent is still in charge and with some issues the parent holds veto power because he or she knows what's best for the child. **Do not use family problem solving unless you really are open to negotiation.**

Teach Family Conflict Management Skills

Family communication and problem-solving skills are essential to family life. There are times, however, when there is so much conflict in a family, that it is impossible to use these valuable skills. In this case, it can be helpful first to use family conflict management skills to calm down and then use family communication and problem-solving skills to solve the problem that created the conflict in the first place.

Step 1: Introduce Family Conflict Management Skills to Family

Again, to accomplish many of these goals, it may be necessary to have a family meeting. Be sure everyone is calm and is OK with being together before attempting such a meeting.

The first task for the family is to recognize the signals that tell them they are experiencing too much conflict. Make sure everyone understands the importance of first recognizing family conflict signals. If you don't recognize family conflict, you can't do anything about it. In this regard, it is helpful to review three different types of family conflict signals: (1) body, (2) thoughts, and (3) actions of self/other. All family members should participate in a discussion to generate examples of signals with someone writing them down.

Some signals that could be discussed include the following:

Body signals	Thought signals	Action signals
• Breathing rate increased	• "She's making me mad."	• Raised voices
• Heart rate increased	• "I hate her!"	• Angry facial expressions
• Sweating increased	• "I wish she were dead."	• Angry body postures
• Face color flushed	• "I'm going to hit her."	• Put-down verbalizations
• Muscle tension increased	• "I wish she would move out of the house."	• Interrupting
• Voice tone raised		

After family members learn how to recognize conflict, they need to learn how to manage it. The most helpful strategy is to separate for a "family cool down." Family cool down involves family members separating from each other for a brief period of time to calm down. Family members should agree ahead of time that any one of them can call a family cool down when someone recognizes that there is family conflict occurring. The family cool down involves separating for some agreed-upon time (e.g., 5 or 10 minutes). While the family members are separated, they practice dealing with their own anger and frustration. This might involve deep breathing, tensing and relaxing muscles, and reciting "helpful self-statements" (e.g., "I'm not going to let her get to me." "I'm going to try and stay cool." "I'll try to say it in a different way to get my point across to her."). After family members have settled down, come back together and use family communication and problem-solving skills. The **Family Cool Down** chart (at the end of the chapter) summarizes all the procedures just discussed. Family members could have one or both of these charts in their hands as they try to solve problems and cope with family conflict.

Step 2: Practice Family Conflict Management Skills

As before, it is helpful to practice these skills with neutral and easy problems before implementing them with difficult problems. To accomplish this, do some role-play exercises with the family, acting out pretend conflict situations. All family members should work together to practice all the skills.

Step 3: Use Family Conflict Management Skills in Real Life

After all members of the family have learned the skills in practice, they can use them when real-life family conflict emerges. It may be difficult, but when family conflict arises, try to go through each step one by one. After the family has cooled off, try to use family communication and problem-solving skills to solve the original problem that caused the conflict. It may be helpful to post the Family Cool Down or **Family Conflict Management** charts (at the end of the chapter) for family members to refer to when conflict arises.

Using All Family Interaction Skills Together

Although we have discussed all of the family interaction skills separately, in actuality they are commonly used together. It might be helpful to post or give family members copies of the charts provided at the end of this chapter to look at as family events unfold. It is conceivable that two or more of the family interaction skills may be needed at the same time. For example, if a parent and a teen get into an argument, they may need to cool down first and then try to solve the problem that created the argument while using good communication skills. Try hard to lead family members to use these skills as needed on an ongoing basis.

LET'S WORK IT OUT

Let's retell the story of Steve, Martha, and Mike: It's a Friday night, and Mike is about to go out for the evening. The following discussion takes place in the family kitchen just before he leaves:

MIKE: I am going to Jeff's house for his birthday party.

STEVE: OK. Be home by 11 o'clock.

MIKE: (*annoyed and voice raised*) You've got to be kidding me! It's Friday and it's Jeff's birthday. I'm not coming in at 11:00. Jeff said his parents will let everyone stay until 1 A.M. Why can't I?

STEVE: (*firm*) Mike, calm down. Let's discuss this.

MIKE: I don't want to discuss it. I'm staying out until 1:00 like everyone else! It's Jeff's birthday!

STEVE: OK, things are getting too hot here. Let's take a 10-minute family cool down and then we'll discuss this.

MIKE: (*sarcastically*) Oh, come on! You have got to be kidding.

MARTHA: Mike, we agreed that we would try to solve our problems a little bit better. Let's all cool down like your father said and then come back and try to discuss it.

MIKE: (*reluctantly*) OK.

    During the 10-minute break, Steve steps outside and takes some deep breaths. Martha thinks about how she can constructively state her thoughts to Mike. Mike watches TV. Then the family comes back together to continue the discussion.

MARTHA: Let's practice communicating while we try to solve this problem. Let's look at the Family Communication Skills chart.

MIKE: Do we have to?

STEVE: Come on. Let's try it. Let's try to use the DOs as we discuss this.

The family goes on to discuss the problem using family communication skills. They agree that the usual curfew will remain 11 o'clock on Friday nights. However, since it is Jeff's birthday, the parents will make an exception and allow Mike to come home at midnight.

FAMILY RELATIONSHIP SUCCESS PLAN 3: DEVELOPING FAMILY ROUTINES AND RITUALS

WHATEVER HAPPENS

Doug and Serena have always approached family life with their daughter Emma in a "whatever happens" kind of way. They are the type of family to eat on the run, get to bed whenever, and let Emma do whatever she wants as long as she is safe. Both parents are busy with work, and Emma has a full schedule of extracurricular activities, including hockey and piano lessons. Doug and Serena usually take turns with caretaking responsibilities pertaining to Emma. Although there is a bond among all of them, they rarely find time to be together as a family unit. It's unusual for the whole family to be together even for a meal.

This somewhat casual approach to family life worked OK when Emma was in preschool and even into her early elementary years. But now Emma is in fourth grade. This year Doug and Serena have been receiving increasing reports from the teacher that Emma is disorganized and frequently off-task, often does not hand in homework assignments, and goofs off a lot, which distracts her classmates. Doug and Serena were talking about Emma the other night and reflected on their family life. They realized that Emma has no real responsibilities at home, that they do not always know if Emma has homework, and there is no consistent bedtime at their house. They wonder if their unstructured lifestyle may be contributing to Emma's school problems.

If families are unorganized and unpredictable the children within them may be too. **Family routines** are essential to family life because they dictate how a family operates. If there are few routines, the family operates loosely and may not accomplish important tasks. Children who grow up in families without routines may have less opportunity to learn how to be organized and get things done.

Family rituals are also important to family life because they provide meaning and a sense of identity among family members. Celebrations, traditions, and ongoing family-focused proceedings such as family dinner time bolster the family. Family rituals can be an anchor for children because they promote a sense of stability and security.

Indeed researchers have determined that families with routines and rituals function better than families without them. In families where there is an emphasis on routines and rituals children have fewer behavioral and adjustment problems and couples report higher marital satisfaction. It seems that developing family routines and rituals enhances family life.

Developing Family Routines

The main idea behind routines is to establish order, predictability, and structure in everyday family life. One way to develop family routines is to **tighten up the daily schedule.** This can be accomplished by setting up a regular schedule including:

- Regular wake up time
- Regular mealtimes (breakfast, lunch, dinner)
- Planned time with friends
- Planned time with family
- Regular shower or bath time
- Regular bedtime

Another routine that is helpful revolves around **responsibilities and expectations for the child,** including:

- Regular chores (e.g., dishes, clean room)
- Regular homework time
- Clean up after yourself
- Take the dog for a walk

The above family routine lists are presented as a beginning point. You can modify and add to them to make it specific to your family.

Developing Family Rituals

Family rituals can be purposefully planned to make sure they occur. The main intent is to set aside time for special family events and make them "institutionalized" within the family. If special family events are repeated in a predictable way, they become an important and valued family activity. Below is a brief list of possible family rituals:

- Regular family meals
- Holidays, birthdays, etc.
- Family traditions
- Cultural and/or religious traditions
- Celebrate successes of family members

The above family ritual list is offered as a staring point. You can modify and add to it to make it specific to your family.

LET'S GET ORGANIZED

With increasing demands on the family as Emma gets older, Doug and Serena realize they need to put a bit more structure into family life. They establish a schedule for Emma that includes doing homework after supper (with parents reviewing what she needs to accomplish) and going to bed by 9:00 each school night. They also institute a policy of Emma assisting with dishes each night and cleaning her room every Saturday. For the foreseeable future, they will check in with Emma's teacher on a weekly basis regarding her general school progress and specific homework assignments that may be due. With their fast-paced lifestyle it is hard to have regular family meals, but they do think that it would be feasible to implement a Sunday afternoon dinner ritual. All family members feel good about these planned routines and rituals, and Doug and Serena are optimistic that this effort will help Emma.

CHARTS FOR CHAPTER 8

FAMILY COMMUNICATION SKILLS

DON'TS

- Long lectures or "sermons"
- Blaming (e.g., "You need to stop
  _____" "It's your fault," etc.)

- Vague statements (e.g., "Shape up," "Knock it off," "I don't like that," etc.)
- Asking negative questions (e.g., "Why do you always do that?", "How many times must I tell you?")
- Poor listening with looking away, silent treatment, crossing arms, and so forth
- Interrupting others

- Not checking to see if you really understand others
- Put-downs (e.g., "You're worthless," "I'm sick of you," etc.), threats, and so forth

- Yelling, screaming, and so forth
- Sarcasm

- Going from topic to topic
- Bringing up old issues, past behavior
- Not matching verbal and nonverbal communications (e.g., saying, "I love you," while pounding one's fist angrily on the table)
- Keeping feelings inside
- Scowling, directing antagonistic facial expressions toward others

- "Mind reading" or assuming you know what other people think

DOs

- Use brief statements of 10 words or less
- Use I statements (e.g., "I feel _____ when _____") or take responsibility for your own actions
- Use direct and specific statements (e.g., "Stop teasing your sister")
- Use direct and specific statements (e.g., "Stop teasing your brother")

- Actively listen with good eye contact, leaning forward, nodding, and so forth
- Let each person completely state his/her thoughts before stating yours
- Give feedback/paraphrase (e.g., restate what another said to you)
- Be constructive (e.g., "I'm concerned about your grades," "Something is bothering me; can we discuss it?", etc.)
- Use a neutral/natural tone of voice
- Say what you mean, be specific and straightforward
- Stay on one topic
- Focus on here and now
- Match verbal and nonverbal communication (e.g., saying "I love you," while smiling)

- Express feelings to others appropriately
- Use appropriate facial expressions toward others
- Really listen to others' point of view; ask questions to make sure you understand

FAMILY PROBLEM SOLVING

1. **Stop!! What is the problem we are having?**
   - Try to avoid blaming individuals.
   - Focus on how family members are interacting and causing problems together.
   - State specifically what the problem is so that everyone agrees.

2. **What are some plans we can use?**
   - Think of as many alternative plans as possible.
   - Don't evaluate or criticize any family member's ideas.
   - Don't discuss any one solution until you have generated many alternatives.

3. **What is the best plan we could use?**
   - Think of what would happen if the family used each of the alternatives.
   - Think about how each alternative would make each family member feel.
   - Decide which alternative is most likely to succeed and make most family members feel OK.
   - Reach an agreement by as many family members as possible.

4. **Do the plan.**
   - Try the plan as best the family can.
   - Don't criticize or say, "I told you so."

5. **Did our plan work?**
   - Evaluate the plan.
   - Determine if everyone is satisfied with the way the problem was solved.
   - If the solution didn't work, repeat the entire family problem-solving process again.

Try to stay focused on the here and now. Do not bring up old issues when trying to do family problem solving.

FAMILY COOL DOWN

1. Are we too angry at each other?

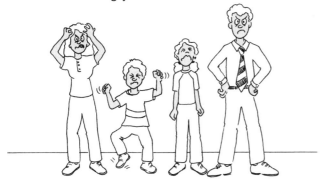

2. Briefly separate to cool down.

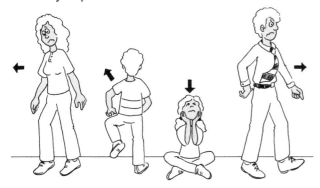

3. Come back together to solve the problem.

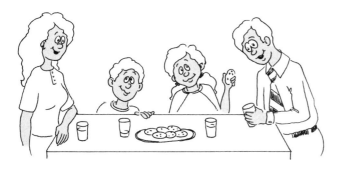

FAMILY CONFLICT MANAGEMENT

1. **Recognizing Conflict**—Each family member learns to recognize when they or others are so angry that effective problem solving and communication are impossible. Family members become aware of escalating anger/conflict signals such as loud voices, angry facial expressions, critical communication, angry thoughts, increased heart and/or breathing rate, increased sweating and/or muscle tension, and so forth.

2. **Coping with Conflict**—The family agrees ahead of time that when they recognize escalating anger/conflict, they will take a previously agreed-upon break (e.g., separate for 10 minutes). Each family member will then try to cope with anger through relaxation and deep breathing, and by utilizing "helpful self-statements" (e.g., "I'm going to try to stay calm," "I'm going to try to think of a better way to get my point across to her," etc.).

3. **Constructive Problem Solving and Communication**—The family reunites and tries to resolve conflicts using family problem-solving and communication skills. Family members try to be assertive, not aggressive, in getting their points across to others.

Chapter 9

Maintaining Improvements for Your Child and Family

Starting something and keeping it going are two very difficult tasks. How often have you made a New Year's resolution? How often have you carried out that New Year's resolution to its completion? Have you ever decided you were going to embark on a diet and exercise program? How successful were you in actually carrying out your health program? It's very difficult to keep something going that is good for you.

By the time you get to this chapter, you very likely have tried to work on one or two Child or Parent or Family Success Plans. Maybe you are beginning to see some progress. The information contained in this book is designed to help you and your child learn skills. The underlying assumption is that by learning these skills, your child's development will be enhanced. Even under the best of circumstances, development unfolds over a long period of time, so **you can expect it will take a long time for your child and family to learn the skills described in this book.** A slow and steady rate of progress makes sense when it comes to skills training. Now that you have started, it is essential to stay the course for the long run so that meaningful gains can be made for your effort.

Getting started is a difficult first step, but keeping it going is equally challenging. Research suggests that many patients do not follow health care regimens prescribed by their physicians. Many patients also fail to follow the treatment plans of mental health providers. Even physicians and mental health providers themselves do not always follow the suggestions and guidelines they give their clients. Indeed, the author of this book doesn't always do what he has written on these pages with his own family!

There is a high probability that you may start out with good intentions but not carry things through because skills are difficult to learn and a struggling child's problems may be ingrained and chronic in nature. Therefore, **it is very important to plan how you will keep it going and maintain improvements once you get started.** What follows are some practical, common-sense suggestions on how you can maintain improvements for you and your child.

PICK THE RIGHT SUCCESS PLAN TO WORK ON

Make sure that you have selected the Success Plan that best matches your child or family's needs and is feasible. Think it through very carefully and select a specific Success Plan to work on. Give it a good effort and try it for a while. Evaluate every now and then how much progress is being made. **If you are satisfied you tried long and hard enough, yet you notice little progress, then it may be time to try something new.** For example, if you try Child Social Success Plan 2, "Teaching a Child Social Problem-Solving Skills" (Chapter 4), but your child is extremely resistant, then perhaps you need to focus on a different skill. You might accomplish a similar objective by instead working with the Family Relationship Success Plan 2 of "Improving Family Interactions" (Chapter 8).

REALISTIC THOUGHTS

Contemporary society seems to be obsessed with quick fixes and cures. We want things to happen yesterday. This is exactly the wrong attitude to have when it comes to trying to learn new skills. These things take time. If you have a realistic attitude at the outset, you're much more likely to be successful. **Sometimes it can take weeks, months, or even years before you see significant changes in your family or child.** Make sure you have realistic expectations for how long it will take for progress to be evident and don't give up if it doesn't happen quickly.

ENLIST THE HELP OF OTHERS

We know that when people tackle a problem together they tend to have more success with whatever task they undertake. People who work together are more likely to stick with exercise routines, quit smoking, or adopt healthy eating habits than individuals who attempt the same agenda alone. This is also true when you try to learn new skills. If you have a spouse or partner available, it may be wise to enlist that person's help in the change process. Try to recruit school personnel to work with your child at the school. Perhaps extended family members could also be of assistance. **Inform these people of the skills that you are working on and try to get them to help you.**

Enlisting help seems to have two effects. First, you will be more likely to stick with the program you started because you have support. Second, you will have some accountability to the other people. They will prompt you and encourage you to stay with it.

GOAL SETTING AND SELF-REINFORCEMENT

It's a good idea to **break a goal down into small, realistic steps.** For example, you may set a goal that you are going to try to teach your child problem-solving skills. A realistic small step toward that goal would be to state that you are going to use problem-solving worksheets with your child for 2 weeks. At the end of 2 weeks, you will evaluate your progress and determine whether you should continue or try something else.

Self-reinforcement involves giving yourself a reward after you've reached your goal. For example, if you were able to use problem-solving worksheets with your child for 2 weeks, you might reward yourself with a special activity or purchase.

PRACTICE SELF-AWARENESS

Sometimes when we set out to change a behavior, we end up continuing the same old behavior anyway, without even realizing it. For example, a dieter reaches for a cookie, eats it, and then realizes what he did. Another example would be the mother who sets out to teach her child problem-solving skills. One day her two sons start a fight about which TV program to watch. This very same mother jumps in and tells her children to take turns watching different shows. Later she realizes she solved a problem for her children that she could have used as an opportunity to teach them how to solve their own problems.

There are several strategies one can use to increase self-awareness. There are numerous charts throughout the book. **Post copies of charts** from this book in strategic locations in your house, such as on the refrigerator or a door. You might also **hang up a sign or signal** somewhere to cue yourself about specific behaviors that you'd like to do. For example, you might put a sign that says "Two-to-One Rule" above the clock in your kitchen. Every time you look at the clock, you will see the sign, which will remind you to make two positive comments to your child for every one instruction or critique you make (see Chapter 8 for more information on the Two-to-One Rule). You could **ask other family members to prompt you** when they notice an opportunity for you to engage in the new behavior. For example, a father might remind a mother not to give in to a child's disobedient behavior and to use time-out instead.

CONDUCT PERIODIC REVIEWS

Review your progress periodically. During these reviews, the goal is to take stock, **evaluate how it's going, and make modifications if needed.** For example, you and your spouse/partner might agree to meet every Sunday evening to review the progress on a specific skill area that you are trying with your child. Write down these periodic review sessions on a calendar.

PLAN FOR RELAPSES

We know that there is a high risk that you and your family will drift back into "old ways." People who are trying to change behaviors frequently have relapses. It is even more likely that relapses will occur when one is dealing with a struggling child who may have chronic problems. How you respond to these relapses is what determines failure or success. You can give up or keep trying to achieve success!

Because relapses are bound to occur, it makes sense to plan ahead for how you will respond to them. The first step is to recognize the signals of relapse. For example, if you notice that your child's behavior problem is getting worse or that you feel under more stress, you may be relapsing. Once you recognize these signals, have a plan of action already in place. Remember that relapses are inevitable, so don't get discouraged. At the point of relapse, you need to gear up and reapply some of the skills that perhaps you have let fall by the wayside. This might entail getting out the charts that you tried several months ago and reusing them.

DON'T GIVE UP

We know that these skills are very difficult to learn and to keep using over time. **If you are consistent and persistent, you will see results.** These skills training procedures fail most often because a parent applies them inconsistently or gives up. Keep trying!

Chapter 10

Accessing Services to Assist the Child and Family

It is possible that even though you have tried several of the Success Plans in this book your child may still need additional support and help. Some children have struggles that are serious enough to warrant mental health, educational, juvenile justice, and/or other community services. This chapter will give parents information about professional help they can obtain to address more serious child and family problems.

Different service systems offer assistance to children and families. The **mental health system** makes treatment available for children with mental health problems typically in a clinical or medical setting. The **educational system** is required to make educational accommodations and special education services available to children with learning and adjustment difficulties that interfere with their ability to profit from school. The **juvenile justice system** attempts to rehabilitate children who have committed a delinquent offense. Finally, the **community provider system** supplies basic family needs and an array of family services for struggling children and their families. In order to access payment for these services through insurance or government funds, a child usually has to qualify by having a specified diagnosis or categorical label. **It is helpful for parents to know the diagnoses and categorical labels that qualify children for services in these systems and what services are available.** By reading this chapter, parents can gain knowledge in order to be better consumers and obtain the best professional help for their struggling child.

OBTAINING HELP IN
THE MENTAL HEALTH SYSTEM

A child must have a mental health diagnosis to qualify for assistance in the mental health system. A **diagnostic assessment** (often with **psychological testing**) is conducted to make a diagnosis. Usually a licensed mental health provider or team of providers conducts an assessment by gathering information from the child, parents, teachers, and others who know the child and uses a variety of different assessment procedures. This often entails an interview with the child and parent(s) and sometimes with educators, social workers, probation officers, or anyone who knows the child well. The interview(s) focus on a review of child symptoms and other potential family and community problems that might be affecting the child. Information about the child's development and the nature of her problem across time is also gathered. Usually the child, parents, and teachers complete questionnaires about the child. Depending on the problems at hand, additional intelligence testing, achievement testing (reading, math, writing, and academic subject knowledge), and neuropsychological testing (memory, attention, and information processing) or medical exams may be administered to the child. Table 10.1 summarizes the typical components of a diagnostic assessment that incorporates psychological testing information.

The *Diagnostic and Statistical Manual of Mental Disorders* (DSM-IV-TR), a diagnostic system published by the American Psychiatric Association in 2000, is utilized to make a diagnosis in a child. DSM-IV-TR provides information regarding all mental heath disorders and explains the symptoms or problems a child must have in order to be given a diagnosis. Mental health professionals take all the information gathered through the diagnostic assessment and use it to derive diagnoses of the child according to DSM-IV-TR criteria. **Please review Chapter 1 for information on the most common DSM-IV-TR diagnoses for a child.**

Once a diagnosis is made, a treatment plan is developed. The mental health provider will offer treatment(s) that match the child's diagnoses and family's needs.

Mental Health Treatments That Work

Psychosocial treatments emphasize skills building similar to that described in preceding chapters of this book. The main difference between the skills building offered in a mental health setting and what is discussed in this book is that a professional practitioner can assist the child and family in learning skills.

TABLE 10.1. Common Diagnostic Assessment and Psychological Evaluation Information

Client description and reason for referral

Sources of information

Presenting problem(s)

Review of functional domains
- Current mental status
- Disruptive behavior disorder symptoms
- Depression symptoms
- Anxiety symptoms
- Social/interpersonal problems
- Learning problems
- Family relationships
- Other problems

Health/medical status
- Past/current medical concerns
- Past/current medications

Developmental history
- Prenatal
- Early development
- Recent development

Family history
- Living arrangements across time
- Divorce, maltreatment/domestic violence, parent personal problems

Educational history
- Special education
- Accommodations

Mental health history
- Child
- Parents/extended family

Chemical health history
- Child
- Parents/extended family

Psychological evaluation results
- Intellectual/neuropsychological/achievement tests
- Personality/psychopathology tests
- Emotional functioning tests
- Parent/teachers rating scales

DSM-IV-TR diagnoses
- Axis I   Clinical disorders
- Axis II   Personality disorders and mental retardation
- Axis III   General medical condition
- Axis IV   Psychosocial and environmental factors
- Axis V   Global assessment of functioning

Conclusions

Recommendations

Treatment plan

Psychosocial treatments are typically delivered to a child and family over approximately 10 to 20 sessions. Follow-up "booster" sessions are usually conducted to make sure the child and family continue making progress. The exact number of sessions can be more or less depending on the presenting problems and severity. **It is important for the child and family to receive the "full dose" of a psychosocial intervention.** In other words, the child and family should attend all of the recommended sessions so that meaningful progress can be made. Unfortunately many families drop out of mental health services prematurely and therefore do not derive the full benefit. It is necessary to attend mental health appointments consistently. **The most common psychosocial interventions are relaxation-based therapies, cognitive-behavioral therapy, social competence training, and parent and family skills training.**

Relaxation-based therapies focus on teaching a child relaxation and general coping skills. These interventions are most often used to treat anxiety disorders in children but are also employed with children who have anger problems. The child is taught relaxation skills and then is exposed to whatever situation or problem is making her feel anxious or upset in a step-by-step fashion. The child is confronted with the anxiety-provoking situation or object first through imagining it and then by actually experiencing it. For example, a child might be anxious about going to school. The child would be taught to relax and imagine getting up in the morning, getting dressed, eating breakfast, and so on until she imagines herself at school. In later sessions the child actually goes to the school setting, first when no one is around, then when just teachers are around, and so on until she is eventually able to go to school. The child is coached to remain calm and relaxed throughout all of these steps.

Cognitive-behavioral therapy is a child-focused skills training procedure that changes unhelpful thinking patterns and improves the child's general coping skills. This type of therapy is most often employed with children who have mood and anxiety disorders. The child learns to identify unhelpful thoughts, understand why the thoughts are unhelpful, and replace them with helpful thoughts that result in positive emotional experiences. Through cognitive-behavioral therapy the child also learns to use "self-talk" (thinking to oneself) to think about her behavior and control emotions such as anger.

Social competence training enhances the child's social behaviors and social problem-solving skills. This particular treatment is used with children who have disruptive behavior disorders and has been tried with children exhibiting mood and pervasive developmental disorders. Usually children are trained in groups and learn how to share, cooperate, and solve social problems. Often a point system of rewards and consequences is used during the group while the children are learning their skills.

A psychosocial intervention commonly used in the mental health setting is **parent and family skills training.** This is a proven treatment that improves child, parent, and family functioning by teaching the parents and family members skills. This particular approach is commonly used with children who have disruptive behavior disorders but is also employed with almost all psychiatric disorders in children. There is strong research support for this approach to treatment. Parents learn to manage their child's behavior, teach their child skills, improve the parent–child relationship, and develop family-wide skills such as conflict resolution and communication. Parent and family skills training should be emphasized in any mental health treatment plan.

Substance abuse treatment is sometimes used for children with substance abuse or dependency problems. Although some would argue that this is not technically a mental health treatment, it is placed in the mental health section of this book because substance abuse and dependence are diagnostic categories in the DSM-IV-TR. The child or teen must participate in an assessment to determine if she qualifies for a substance-related diagnosis. Since many substance abusers minimize or deny their use, it is important to obtain information from a variety of sources such as parents, friends, teachers, and so on.

Once diagnosed, a substance abuse treatment approach needs to be selected based on severity of substance abuse. **Outpatient programs** are used for the least severe substance abusers and involve weekly office visits, usually delivered within a group treatment format. **Short-term inpatient programs** are for moderately severe substance abusers. Patients usually are admitted to short-term inpatient programs for about 30 days. **Long-term residential programs** are for the most severe substance abusers, who have often already tried and failed with less restrictive approaches. All of these programs provide increasingly intensive interventions usually emphasizing education, skills training, and family interventions. Some programs also incorporate the 12-step philosophy. Research reveals that many substance abusers relapse, but eventually derive benefit with continued treatments.

Psychiatric medications are commonly administered to children diagnosed with mental health problems. These medications affect the production of neurotransmitters in the central nervous system including serotonin, norepinephrine, and dopamine. The neurons in the central nervous system either produce more, or are more receptive to, certain neurotransmitters when affected by the medications. There are several classes of medications that are commonly prescribed by physicians to treat children with mental health problems. The most commonly used medication class is the **stimulants.** Stimulant medications improve symptoms of ADHD, including inattention, hyperactivity, and impulsivity, and to some extent reduce aggression. **Strattera** is a nonstimulant medication that is used effectively in treating symptoms of ADHD. There are four broad types of **antidepressant** medications: tricyclic, selective serotonin reuptake inhibitors (SSRIs), monamine oxidase inhibitors (MAOIs), and atypical antidepressants. The antidepressants help children with depression and anxiety and are somewhat helpful in reducing aggressive behavior as well. **Mood stabilizers** are used for children who have bipolar disorder and/or severe aggression. **Antihypertensive** medications are prescribed to treat significant anger, aggression, and resistant ADHD symptoms in children. **Anxiolytic** medications help children who are suffering from anxiety. The **typical and atypical antipsychotic** medications are effective in treating children with psychosis or with severe anger and aggression.

In clinical practice **medications are often combined** to treat comorbid or multiple problem areas in children. The decision to medicate a child should be made carefully after much deliberation. Usually the physician will slowly adjust the dosage level of the chosen medication until the child achieves maximum clinical benefit with minimal side effects. The physician should monitor the child while the child is on the medications to determine whether or not they are effective and to guard against side effects. Not all children are "responders" to medications. Sometimes it is necessary to adjust the dosage or type of medication. Finally, it is critical that any medications taken by a child conform to the doctor's prescribed dose and schedule for as long as is advised to derive optimal effects.

Parents should be aware of what is known about the effects of medications on children. The most research exists evaluating the stimulants, with less research available regarding the effects of the other medications described above. Little controlled research has been conducted evaluating the effects of medications on preschoolers, although several large-scale studies are currently underway. In addition, only three stimulants (Adderall, Concerta, and Ritalin), one nonstimulant (Strattera), and one antidepressant (Prozac) have been approved for use in children by the United States Food and Drug Administration. The other above-mentioned medications are prescribed routinely using "off label" prescription practices, which means that physicians can use medications for other than approved purposes using good professional judgment and carefully monitoring the situation. It is recommended that parents become well educated about medications for children and consult with a knowledgeable physician.

Another area of mental health services relates to the setting in which they are provided and how intensive they are. Increasingly **restrictive mental health**

settings are used to stabilize and treat children and teens displaying increasingly severe levels of symptoms. Most mental health services are delivered in an outpatient setting where the child meets with a therapist and/or physician on a regular basis. If the child's symptoms are severe enough, she might qualify for day treatment or partial hospitalization in which case the child spends the day in a controlled mental health setting. Unfortunately some children require hospitalization or residential treatment if their symptoms and problems are severe and/or they are considered a danger to self or others.

OBTAINING HELP IN THE EDUCATIONAL SYSTEM

Federal laws require the educational system to provide services for children who have emotional, behavioral, or learning problems that limit their ability to succeed in school. To qualify for such services children need to be labeled according to educational categories. To obtain a categorical label, a team of educational professionals, including teachers, social workers, school psychologists, speech and language clinicians, occupational therapists, and outside consultants, often evaluates the child. These professionals use observations, testing, and interviews to conduct an assessment. The professional team combine their results to determine the child's needs and resulting interventions or services.

Educational Categories for Entitled Services

This section will review educational categories that are commonly assigned to struggling children in schools. These are legal designations that qualify children for accommodations and services so they can succeed at school. There are two special education categories. The first special education category is **Learning Disability,** which is used when a child exhibits reading, written language, or arithmetic skills that are markedly below expectations given that child's intellectual abilities and when compared to same-age or grade peers. The second special education category is that of **Emotional Behavioral Disorder,** which is reserved for a child exhibiting social, emotional, and behavioral problems interfering with her accomplishment of educational and social tasks in the school environment. More often than not a child with Emotional Behavioral Disorder also qualifies for a DSM-IV-TR diagnosis in the mental health system.

Two other disability-based categories also entitle children to assistance at school. The category of **Other Health Impaired** is based on the concept of a medical disability. The child may have a learning or developmental disability, mental retardation, speech and language difficulty, or hearing or visual difficulty that compromises her schooling. A **504 plan** is for children with "special needs" that interfere with their capacity to learn at school. Special needs of students include physical, emotional, or psychiatric disability. It should be noted that the diagnosis of ADHD qualifies for school-based accommodations under the Other Health Impaired or 504 categories. Other, less common categories of child problems exist that will help a child obtain assistance at school. The educational professionals at your child's school will be able to help pinpoint the best category for your struggling child.

Educational Services

School personnel will devise an **Individualized Education Plan (IEP)** for a child who qualifies for services. The IEP specifies a plan targeting a child's unique academic and/or emotional/behavioral needs and is used to organize school services for the child. The IEP describes the nature of the child's learning, emotional, or behavioral problem(s) and states goals and objectives. Specific target behaviors and corresponding interventions are noted. Accommodations and/ or special education services are then offered to the child. The school, parents, and child work together in developing and implementing the IEP.

School services are provided to children based on the concept of **"least restrictive environment."** School officials attempt to work with the child in a less restrictive environment providing less intensive services first, followed by a more restrictive environment and more intensive services later if needed. A child will usually first receive assistance in her mainstream classroom. If this does not work, then she might be referred for special assistance outside of the classroom, and at the most restrictive level, into a self-contained classroom or specialized school.

The least restrictive services involve working with the child and/or teacher in the child's classroom. **Academic skills building** interventions teach the child skills such as staying on task, organization, study habits, and so on. These are used with children displaying Learning Disability and, to some extent, Emotional Behavior Disorder. Some children receive **tutoring and direct instruction** in an academic subject (such as reading). Occasionally specific **accommodations** are made that account for a child's disability such as extra time to complete schoolwork or materials presented visually instead of verbally. **Classroom behavior management** strategies are also commonly used and can be very effective. This has to do with the teacher providing rewards and consequences depending on the child's behavior in the classroom. A very powerful intervention is **home–school notes** to improve communication between home and school about the child's progress. These procedures are usually enough to help most struggling children.

Special education is reserved for children who are categorized as having a Learning Disability and/or Emotional Behavior Disorder at a more severe level. Special education services can range from consulting with a teacher to placing the child in a self-contained classroom. The levels of restriction and intensity of the services are dependent on the severity of the child's difficulty and how she responded to less intensive interventions previously. Many of the strategies discussed in the preceding paragraph are made available to the child in a more concentrated manner through special education.

OBTAINING HELP
IN THE JUVENILE JUSTICE SYSTEM

The mandate of the juvenile justice system is to rehabilitate "juvenile delinquents" and keep citizens safe from those who cannot be rehabilitated. **Delinquency** is a legal designation given to a child or teen who has committed a crime and is now within the juvenile court's jurisdiction. A child or teen enters the juvenile justice system by committing a misdemeanor or felony criminal offense. If the child ends up in juvenile court, a probation officer or case manager is typically assigned to work with the child and family. Federal law dictates that states and counties must provide an array of services for juvenile delinquents.

Through either informal means or by court order, the juvenile delinquent can be required to participate in different types of interventions. **Diversion** is used for low-risk delinquents who have good potential to change. This could involve the juvenile participating in services such as classes for shoplifters, community programming (e.g., after-school activities, sports, arts, music), and/or performance of restitution. Through restitution the juvenile offender pays back the community or the victim by performing community service or making monetary reimbursement. **Probation** is in essence a form of monitoring and accountability to make the juvenile delinquent follow rules and access needed services. The court might direct the delinquent to attend school, obey curfew and home rules, and/or abstain from drug or alcohol use. The probation officer monitors the delinquent to make sure she follows through and reports to the court about her progress. **Rehabilitation** can include the above interventions and, where applicable, the treatment of the juvenile delinquent's underlying mental health, medical, or chemical dependency problems. Participation in these services might also be part of a probation requirement. **Confinement,** or incarceration, is reserved for those who have committed serious felony criminal acts. Those individuals are confined for punishment and sometimes because they are deemed a potential danger to society.

OBTAINING HELP IN COMMUNITY SYSTEMS

Various community programs offer services for high-risk children and families. Often a local county-funded system of care is mandated to provide services through for-profit and nonprofit community agencies. Frequently, to qualify, a child must live in a specific geographic area where the services are provided and/or be labeled with **Severe Emotional Disturbance.** The Severe Emotional Disturbance designation is used by states to qualify children for state-funded mental health and community services. Children with Severe Emotional Disturbance have emotional and behavioral disorders (usually a DSM-IV-TR category) that are severe and place them at high risk for needing restrictive intensive mental health services or out-of-home placement. The Severe Emotional Disturbance label can be utilized by parents to obtain state- and county-funded community-based services for a child.

The community system provides community- and home-based interventions. **In-home therapeutic services** addressing a child's mental health and/or family problems can be quite effective. This entails a mental health provider going into the home to provide direct service to the child and family in an intensive manner. Through **family support case management** a case manager works with the family by providing practical support and assistance in obtaining additional services to help them (e.g., housing, job training, medical services, etc.). **Mentoring and after-school programs** expose a child to positive adults, peers, and activities that they can "bond" to in the community. Sometimes a **"wraparound"** concept is utilized where a case manager attempts to connect the child and family to a variety of mental health, education, and community services (see next section for more details).

COORDINATED SERVICES APPROACHES

A **Coordinated Services** approach may ultimately be best for children and families with more severe problems. This approach involves provision of multiple services to address multiple child and family problems. If needed, it is best to participate in two or more mental health, educational, juvenile justice, and community services at the same time.

In Chapter 1 we reviewed the array of risk and assets/protective factors that influence children's development. Those risk and assets/protective factors can be best addressed if a parent conducts child- and family-focused skills training like what was described earlier in this book and makes sure the child gets all mental health, educational, juvenile justice, and community services that she might need. A coordinated services approach will ultimately be the best way to help a struggling child to succeed.

Coordinated Services can be organized informally by a parent or formally by a case manager. Parents can review all the information in this chapter to get ideas on how to access services in various systems of care and then advocate for their child to obtain these services. If the child has been determined to have Severe Emotional Disturbance (see preceding section), she may qualify for a local county-funded **mental health or child welfare case manager.** This individual will know local resources and be adept at organizing and delivering a continuum of services for the child and family.

PRACTITIONER'S GUIDE

Chapter 11

A Practitioner's Guide to Using This Book with Children and Parents

This chapter provides guidelines for practitioners using this book, hereafter referred to as the "Skills Training" book, in their work with children and families. This includes a review of general parameters for conducting parent- and child-focused skills training interventions, as well as specific ideas for incorporating the Skills Training book into a practitioner's intervention efforts with a particular child and family. A parent may also benefit from reading this chapter to gain an increased understanding of the foundation on which the procedures and methods described in earlier chapters are built.

REVIEW OF SKILLS TRAINING LITERATURE

The instructions provided in earlier chapters of this book are derived from research-supported Parent and Family Skills Training and child-focused Social Competence Training programs aimed primarily at children with behavior problems and their families. This section will present a brief review of this literature. See Bloomquist and Schnell (2002) and the citations below for a thorough discussion.

Parent and family skills training (PFST) involves practitioners teaching parents and family members skills that enhance child, parent, and fam-

ily functioning. Research-supported PFST programs include *Parent Training* (Patterson, 1975; Patterson, Cobb, & Ray, 1973; Patterson, Reid, Jones, & Conger, 1975), *Helping the Noncompliant Child* (McMahon & Forehand, 2003), *Incredible Years* (parent component) (Webster-Stratton, 1992, 1996; Webster-Stratton & Reid, 2003), *Parent–Child Interaction Therapy* (Brinkmeyer & Eyberg, 2003; Eyberg & Boggs, 1998; Eyberg, Boggs, & Algina, 1995), *Parent Management Training* (Kazdin, 2003), *Defiant Child and Defiant Teen Programs* (Anastopoulas, Shelton, DuPaul, & Guevremont, 1993; Barkley, 1997; Barkley, Edwards, & Robin, 1999; Barkley, Edwards, Laneri, Fletcher, & Metevia, 2001), *Triple P—Positive Parenting Program* (Sanders 1999), *Problem Solving and Communications Skills Training* (Robin & Foster, 1989), *Adolescent Transitions Program* (Dishion & Kavanagh, 2003), and *Multisystemic Therapy* (Henggeler & Lee, 2003; Henggeler, Schoenwald, Borduin, Rowland, & Cunningham, 1998). What these PFST approaches have in common (to varying degrees) is a focus on training parents in child management and parent–child bonding strategies, addressing parents' personal problems through coping skills training, and improving family-wide interactions by training family members in specified family skills.

A significant amount of research has been conducted evaluating PFST. Each of the above cited PFST programs has supporting research to suggest it is effective (see citations for details). General conclusions can be made about the effectiveness of PFST by examining reviews of the literature in this area. Whether it is meta-analysis (Serketich & Dumas, 1996) or narrative reviews (Kazdin, 1997, 2003; Brestan & Eyberg, 1998), PFST has been found to be quite effective. It has been shown to improve child and parent functioning, parenting skills, and family interactions. The research reveals that PFST not only achieves statistical significance, but also "clinical significance" where scores on indicators of child and family functioning are in the "normal" range after PFST. The outcomes for PFST are somewhat better for preschool/school-age children than for teens. Multisystemic and family-focused skills interventions work best with teenagers (e.g., Barkley et al., 2001; Dishion & Kavanagh 2003; Henggeler et al., 1998). Negative outcomes, such as drop out and lack of progress, are seen in a small percentage of families who usually have the most severe level of problems to begin with (Assemany & McIntosh, 2002).

Common practice guidelines can be derived by looking for procedural similarities across the aforementioned PFST programs. Effective practitioners working with families using PFST form good relationships with parents and children and actively lead family members to develop new skills. Good results in PFST are accomplished when practitioners utilize behavioral training procedures such as instruction, modeling (including video modeling), role playing, practice, feedback, reinforcement, and homework exercises. Interventions are delivered in small groups or with individual families. Approximately 10 to 18 sessions are utilized, although the number of sessions is adjusted to allow for families who learn at different paces (up to 50 sessions for some families). Usually two to six sessions are utilized to train any one particular skill (e.g., two sessions for time-out or five sessions for family communication skills). Follow-up booster sessions are recommended so that families maintain progress. The common content of what is taught in PFST is detailed in Table 11.1. This same PFST content is integrated into the Skills Training book. Instead of a practitioner teaching the parent and family, however, the parent is taught these skills by following the instructions in the book.

Social competence training (SCT) refers to methods used by practitioners to teach children skills to enhance their social-emotional developmental competence. Although practitioner-led SCT is not promoted in the Skills Training book, that literature nonetheless informs the methods described there because the book explains to parents how they can teach similar skills to their child. Research-validated SCT programs include *Social Behavior Training* (Bierman, Greenberg, & Conduct Problems Prevention Research Group, 1996), *Prosocial Coping Skills Training* (Prinz, Blechman, & Dumas, 1994), *Promoting Alternative Thinking Strategies Program* (Greenberg, Kusche, Cook, & Quamma, 1995; Kam, Greenberg, & Kusche, 2003), *Attribution Retraining Program* (Hudley et al., 1998; Hudley & Graham, 1993), *Self-Management Training* (Hinshaw, 2000; Hinshaw, Henker, & Whalen, 1984a, 1984b), *Verbal Self-Instruction Training* (Kendall & Braswell, 1993), *Problem-Solving Training* (Kazdin, 2003), *Anger Coping and Coping Power Training* (Larsen & Lochman, 2002; Lochman, Barry, & Pardini, 2003), *Second Step Program* (Frey, Hirschstein, & Guzzo, 2000; Grossman et al., 1997), and *Incredible Years* (child component) (Webster-Stratton, 1996; Webster-Stratton & Reid, 2003). What these SCT programs have in common (to varying degrees) is the shaping of a child's positive behavior and teaching him or her social behavior, social cognitive, and emotion regulation skills.

A fair amount of research has been conducted to determine the effects of SCT. Each of the above cited SCT programs has supporting research to suggest it is effective (see citations for details). General conclusions can be made about the efficacy of SCT by examining reviews of the literature in this area. Inspection of meta-analysis (Beelman, Pfingsten, & Losel, 1994; Quinn, Kavele, Mathur, Rutherford, & Forness, 1999) and narrative reviews (Brestan & Eyberg, 1998; McFayden-Ketchum & Dodge, 1998; Taylor, Eddy, & Biglan, 1999) shows that SCT has some research support. Children's behavior and social skills typically improve, but the improvements are often not clinically

TABLE 11.1. Summary of Best Practices Training Content Areas for Parent and Family Skills Training

Training content areas	Best practice
Observing and tracking child behavior	Teach parents to define and pinpoint specific child behaviors; plan when to observe the child; count the frequency of the behavior during child observations.
Encourage child-directed interaction and play	Teach parents to increase relationship enhancing behaviors and decrease relationship detracting behaviors during child-directed play and activities.
Shaping positive behavior with positive attention and reinforcement	Teach parents to increase attention and reinforcement for prosocial child behavior.
Ignoring mild negative behavior	Teach parents to reduce attention for mild child problem behaviors.
Defusing power struggles	Teach parents stress management skills to stay calm and use common-sense strategies to avoid and defuse escalating child behavior.
Using time-out/removal of privileges for noncompliance	Teach parents to stay calm and use effective commands/warning/time-out or removal of privileges when rules are violated.
Using standing or house rules for behavior	Teach parents to state the rules explicitly and use time-out or removal of privileges when rules are violated.
Using token system for behavior management	Teach parents to use tokens/points to shape child behavior.
Monitoring and supervising children	Teach parents to keep track of children; provide structure and expectations.
Addressing parents' personal and other family problems	Teach family members to use common-sense/practical strategies to deal with personal, parent/family, and contextual problems; teach them skills to cope with stress, restructure unhelpful thoughts, and improve marital/family interactions.
Integrating parent and family skills training	Combine multiple skills training content areas into one intervention.

Note. From Bloomquist and Schnell (2002). Copyright 2002 by The Guilford Press. Reprinted by permission.

meaningful. The children may have benefited, but many still have social adjustment problems after SCT. Many authors suggest that SCT should be one component of a multicomponent intervention that also includes work with a child's parents and family. This is especially true if working with a child exhibiting behavior problems.

Common practice guidelines can be derived by looking for procedural similarities across the aforementioned SCT programs. Practitioners who are successful in teaching children social competence skills are enthusiastic and are able to establish good relationships with them. Training is typically conducted within the context of small groups. Sometimes "normal" peers are enrolled in the SCT program to provide examples of adaptive behavior. Practitioners utilize instruction, modeling (including video modeling), role playing, practice, feedback, reinforcement, and homework to teach children skills. Typically group rules are established, and behavioral procedures such as tokens/points systems and time-out are used to manage behavior in the sessions. Approximately 18 to 22 sessions of 40 to 120 minutes are utilized in SCT training. Engaging training materials such as games, puppets, and books are often employed to facilitate training. The common content for SCT programming is presented in Table 11.2. This same SCT content is integrated into the Skills Training book. Instead of the practitioner teaching the child, however, the parent is instructed to assume the lead role in teaching the child.

The Skills Training book offers guidelines that are informed by evidence-based PFST and SCT programs, but also incorporates knowledge in child development/developmental psychopathology and procedural refinements derived from the author's skills training work with many families. The goals and targets of the Skills Training book are similar to those described above for PFST and SCT. Delivery and content practice procedures were extracted from these programs and integrated into the Skills Training book to make available a flexible and individualized approach to help children and families. The skills training procedures are designed to provide explicit training that promotes the child's development. All of the procedures have been field tested over many years within the context of the author's clinical- and research-based service delivery activities. Although the Skills Training book has not been subjected to research evaluation, it nonetheless is empirically, theoretically, and experientially informed.

As mentioned above, the Skills Training book teaches parents skills to enhance their child's developmental status and improve parent/family functioning. **The parent may be assisted in this skills development endeavor by working with a practitioner.** The remainder of this chapter describes how

TABLE 11.2. Summary of Best Practices Training Content Areas for Social Competence Training

Training content areas	Best practices
Social behavior and communication skills training	Teach children observable prosocial behaviors and verbal and nonverbal communication skills.
Affective education	Teach children to identify and label feeling states in self and others.
Social perspective-taking training	Teach children to infer others' thoughts/feelings.
Attribution retraining	Teach children to determine others' intentions and to interpret situations accurately.
Self-monitoring and self-evaluation training	Teach children to accurately observe and evaluate own behavior.
Verbal self-instruction training	Teach children to use internal private speech to regulate behavior.
Problem-solving skills training	Teach children to use methodical steps to solve interpersonal problems.
Anger management training	Teach children to recognize and cope with angry feelings and reactions.
Combining social competence	Combine multiple social competence training content areas into one intervention.

Note. From Bloomquist and Schnell (2002). Copyright 2002 by The Guilford Press. Reprinted by permission.

practitioners can use this book in their work with struggling children and their families.

CREDENTIALS AND CHARACTERISTICS OF AN EFFECTIVE PRACTITIONER

A practitioner is defined here as a service provider within a mental health, educational, juvenile justice, or community setting who serves children and families. Typically practitioners who work with families within those settings have a minimum of a Master's Degree in a human services or educational field and are licensed within their area of professional specialty. Sometimes advanced-degree-seeking trainees or paraprofessionals with a Bachelor's Degree will provide direct service to families under the supervision of a more experienced professional.

Although the individual's credentials are important, they may be less significant than are the personal characteristics of the person and the specific training he or she has received. Many of the PFST and SCT programs reviewed earlier specify the qualities of practitioners who are adept at delivering skills training. First, effective practitioners are good at forming a relationship or connection with a child and family. They are accepting, empathetic, humorous, and are good at communication. Second, effective practitioners are structured and active during the sessions. They are collaborative and guide family members in figuring out what they need to work on, then help them develop and carry out a plan. They are goal oriented and use behavioral training strategies to teach skills (see "Training Methods" section later in this chapter). Finally, it is imperative that a practitioner who delivers skills training to families be trained and receive good supervision. The practitioner should be judged by his or her supervisor as proficient in family-focused skills training methods prior to independent practice.

It seems plausible that effective practitioners using the Skills Training book in their work with families would have a similar professional background and personal characteristics to those described above. Parents who are looking for practitioners to assist their family would be wise to find one with the credentials and characteristics described above.

DETERMINING THE FUNCTIONAL NEEDS OF THE CHILD AND FAMILY

The intervention offered to a child and family ideally will be tailored to their specific needs. It is recommended that a functional needs assessment be conducted before an intervention commences. In this book a functional assessment has to do with **determining the child's developmental status, the nature of the parent or parents' personal well-being, and the quality of family relationships.**

The functional assessment must be undertaken in order to figure out which skills training procedures (Success Plans) will be emphasized with a particular family. Chapters 1 and 2 present information and procedures that can be utilized to conduct functional assessments in important child and parent/family areas. It is best if the practitioner assesses functional status in collaboration with the parents (sometimes involving an older child/teen) by reviewing Chapters 1 and 2 together. In particular, the target characteristic information in Chapter 1, along with the developmental information and parent-ratings in Chapter 2, can serve as a springboard for discussion to determine what areas should be focused on with that particular family. After an area of focus is determined, it is necessary to **specify a corresponding Success Plan** that will be introduced to help the child and/or family to make progress. This is covered at the end of Chapter 2.

PREPARATION FOR CHANGE

Before and during skills training, it is important to make sure the family is prepared to change, thereby increasing the probability that skills training will ultimately succeed. **Preparation for change involves motivating the family, especially the parents, and removing barriers and obstacles that could impede skills training.** The parent receives most of the focus here because it is the parent who will be responsible for the lion's share of the work in implementing any of the procedures described in the Skills Training book. **Preparing the parents and family for change is rooted in a collaborative process between the practitioner and the family.** Collaboration involves forming a cooperative partnership with parents and family members in order to develop and carry out a skills training plan.

Assessing the Family's Readiness for Change

It is imperative to **ascertain the family's "readiness for change."** This is a practitioner's judgment call about the family in terms of problem severity and the parent's capacity to complete the intervention. **Problem severity** means determining the intensity of the child's and family's difficulties, which can range from low to high. Problem severity includes, but is not limited to, the nature of the child's developmental struggles and the family's challenges in day-to-day functioning. The **parent's capacity to complete the intervention** is about the parent's willingness and ability to cooperate and fully participate with an intervention, which can also range from low to high. It includes examining the parent's attitudes about child, self, the recommended intervention, personal problems/strengths, aptitude, and motivation, as well as potential obstacles such as transportation difficulties, not having enough time, and too many everyday life stressors.

Figure 11.1 organizes the family's problem severity and the parent's capacity to complete the intervention into four different quadrants. These four

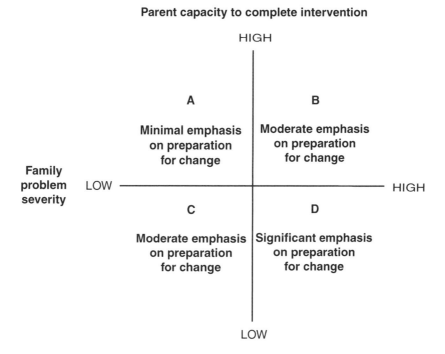

FIGURE 11.1. Family readiness for change and corresponding emphasis on preparation for change.

quadrants can be used to think about a family in terms of needed preparation for change efforts (described below). Families who exhibit low problem severity and high parent capacity to complete the intervention will require minimal emphasis on preparation for change. Families who are high in problem severity and parent capacity to complete the intervention or low in problem severity and parent capacity to complete the intervention will require moderate emphasis on preparation for change. Those families who are exhibiting a high level of problems and low parent capacity to complete the intervention will require maximum preparation for change efforts.

One final caveat as it relates to determining a family's readiness to change. Some children and families have needs so great that they cannot profit from a skills training intervention. **There are several exclusionary criteria that a practitioner should consider that might indicate skills training would be either insufficient or perhaps inappropriate.** These exclusionary criteria include extreme levels of child behavior problems (e.g., repeatedly violent behavior), mental retardation/organic difficulties or psychosis within the child, extreme marital/partner problems or parental psychopathology, and/or a history of child abuse/neglect. If all or some of these exclusionary criteria exist in a particular case, then other interventions might be indicated (see Chapter 10), or the skills training approach might only serve as one facet of an overall comprehensive intervention. In these instances a family will not be ready to adopt new family skills until these serious family issues are addressed.

It is important to understand the family's readiness for change so that preparation for change efforts can be calibrated accordingly. Preparation for change involves enhancing the parent's motivation or "ownership" of the intervention and minimizing potential barriers and obstacles that might derail the skills training effort.

Enhancing Parents' Motivation for Skills Training

It is vital that a parent understands and agrees with the recommended course of action put forth by a practitioner. Parents need to endorse and accept the planned intervention. If that plan includes skills training, they really need to think that skills training is a great idea and be highly motivated to put forth the effort needed to do it right.

Explain Everything

The first step in enhancing parental motivation is to thoroughly **explain all assessment results and recommendations.** For example, if you are a mental health practitioner you would need to explain any DSM-IV-TR diagnoses determined from a diagnostic assessment and review the prognosis and treatment options. Next fully inform family members about a variety of intervention options that are available to them. The practitioner should fully explain the skills training approach, and discuss additional interventions including medications and school- and community-based services. Family members, especially parents, should understand all available intervention options and see how skills training fits into the big picture of a comprehensive intervention plan.

Promote a Developmental Conceptualization of Problems

It is also important to **guide parents to think of their child's problems in developmental terms and explain the development enhancement rationale for skills training.** Have the parents review Chapter 2 and ask them to pinpoint where they think their child is in terms of self-control, social, emotional, and academic development. Explain that children may be chronologically at one stage, but psychologically at another stage (often younger). For example, a child might be 12 years old, but developmentally may be much younger in self-control development in view of the fact he infrequently follows adults' directives or rules at home and school. Once the parents have determined the developmental level of their child, they can then examine their own personal well-being and the quality of their family's relationships that influence their child's development. Thoroughly explain the four domains of childhood development and related parent/family factors (see Chapter 2), and that the goal of the intervention is to get the child back on track developmentally and improve the family. Make sure the parents understand the developmental underpinning of the Skills Training book and that resulting skills training will take a lot of time and effort (i.e., it takes time to facilitate development).

Pick the Right Skills (Success Plan)

Collaborate with the family in choosing an area of focus and determining which Success Plan to implement. This can be accomplished by emphasizing the self-evaluation process described in Chapter 2. Have parents (and older children/teens) rate the six common areas of focus for the child and family and then rank them in order of importance. Ask them to select a Success Plan to make improvements in an identified area of focus. If there is disagreement among family members, keep dialoguing with them about pros and cons of different areas of focus and the corresponding Success Plan(s) until a consensus is reached.

Although it is essential to collaborate with parents, **the practitioner should lead them so they can choose skills training approaches that can be most realistically accomplished.** A practitioner will inevitably come across parents who rate many or all of the six areas of focus as significant problems. When this happens, the practitioner needs to lead the parents in the right direction. A rule of thumb is to focus on salient parent and family variables before focusing on the child. When it comes to the child, it is essential first to make sure the child is compliant and following rules before facilitating his developmental competencies. A child's developmental level should also be considered in selecting an area of focus. The Success Plans relating to problem solving, anger management, and helpful thinking require the child to possess abstract thinking skills. These Success Plans should not be chosen for younger children who may not have the cognitive capacity to benefit from them.

Modify Unhelpful Parent Thoughts about the Intervention and Who Needs to Change

Occasionally parents will doubt the usefulness of a suggested Success Plan. The most common refrain is "we tried that, and it didn't work." The practitioner should carefully discuss what they tried and how they tried it. **Chances are that whatever was previously tried was not executed very well.** For example, a parent may state that he or she has tried time-out with the child, but it didn't work. Most often, parents are inconsistent or give up while applying a particular skill or procedure, and then they deem it ineffective. In these instances it is helpful to discuss the preferred way of executing whatever Success Plan is being suggested and make sure parents understand that skills training only works if parents apply it consistently and persistently (see Chapter 9 for related suggestions).

Sometimes parents have unhelpful beliefs about who needs to change. If a parent blames the child or a spouse/partner/teacher for the problems, then a skills training approach involving that parent will be less likely to work. The practitioner should spend some time before attempting skills training to **make sure the parent at least holds a shared sense of responsibility for many of the problems and, more important, for the solutions.** If the parent expects the child or someone else to do all the changing, then a parent-focused skills training intervention may not be effective. The parent has to commit to the change process before change can really occur.

Cognitive reframing techniques can be used to help parents see their role in the problem. For example, a common statement practitioners hear from parents of a noncompliant child is something like "He's a brat." A statement like that implies the child is the cause of the problem and therefore should be the focus of the intervention. Most practitioners realize they will not get too far intervening with a noncompliant child without involving the parent, but if the parent views the child as the problem, the practitioner may not get far working with the parent. Cognitive reframing might help in this instance. The practitioner could begin cognitive reframing by asking the parent to describe an example of when the child is behaving like a "brat." The parent may say, "I tell him to do something, and he refuses." The practitioner could then reframe the problem by stating something like: "So, there really are two issues here as you describe them. One is you tell him to do something, and the other is he refuses. Let's discuss the way you tell him to do things as the first issue, and then how he refuses. We may need to change how you tell him to do things *and* improve his doing things that you tell him. What do you think?" In this example, the problem has been reframed as involving both the parent and child. Ideally this will help the parent be more receptive to subsequent discussions of parent-focused skills training methods for dealing with a noncompliant child.

Practitioners can also assist family members in accepting shared responsibility for problems by examining in-session family member behavior. For example, parents and teens often blame each other for family disputes and conflicts. As the practitioner sits with the family, invariably a dispute or conflict will occur in a session. The practitioner can then reframe the problem by pointing out how their behavioral responses to each other during the session fueled the conflict. The practitioner could use this example to help family members see that they all have a role in the problem. Family members may then be more receptive to subsequent discussions about family interaction skills training.

Reducing Barriers and Obstacles

No matter how good the practitioner and the intervention plan, if the parents or the family unit is overwhelmed by stressors or burdened by the requirements of the intervention itself, not much change will take place. It is important to reduce barriers and obstacles that could impede progress, so the family will attend and get a "full dose" of the intervention.

Reduce Access Barriers

A family cannot make use of skills training if they cannot access it. For families that have limited resources, this could mean **overcoming the potential barrier of the family not being able to get to skills training sessions.** It may be necessary to deliver skills training in a school or community center or provide transportation to the practitioner's office. To encourage families who have all sorts of pressures, it may be wise to provide food and fun social activities along with skills training when they do show up. It may also be necessary to supply child care for siblings and other children the parents are responsible for.

If the family can't get to you, then consideration should be given to going to the family. It can be quite effective to conduct skills training during in-home visits.

Provide Practical Family Support

Many families who seek help are confronted with significant and multiple stressors. Those problems might include financial tribulations, child abuse/neglect, domestic violence, parent personal problems, and/or a high frequency of stressful life events such as multiple deaths in the family, changing residence frequently, or divorce/separation. It will be quite challenging to conduct skills training with families facing these circumstances. These problems are potentially major obstacles to successful implementation of skills training. In these cases, the family needs a lot of practical support. **It may be necessary to refer a parent or family member to mental health, chemical health, and/or community or social services.** It may be wise to conduct traditional individual/family therapy or refer for medications before conducting skills training. The family may need assistance obtaining basic needs such as housing, food, shelter, and the like. Often other problems are more pressing than the need for skills training. If these problems are not addressed first, or at least simultaneously, there will be little success in skills training. Highly stressed families can benefit from skills training as long as it is combined with other needed and practical strategies.

Facilitate Completion of Homework

In skills training interventions, completion of homework is critical in family members learning and actually using new skills in the home environment. Unfortunately there is often a high rate of noncompliance with homework activities. Throughout this book, attempts have been made to make homework assignments very easy to understand and implement (e.g., charts at the end of each chapter). This should make it a little easier to implement homework assignments. It still will be necessary for the practitioner to **actively monitor the family members' progress with homework and make adjustments when necessary** to enable success with homework.

    When homework noncompliance occurs, it can be useful to discuss obstacles interfering with homework completion. The practitioner could inquire as to whether the skill targeted in the homework exercise was really the best area to focus on. For example, a parent decides to use a Daily Behavior Chart (Chapter 3) with her child, but doesn't. The practitioner could inquire as to whether improving the child's rule-following behavior via behavioral contract was the best area to focus on. If the parent says, "Maybe not," perhaps the practitioner and parent should review other potential target areas of focus in a collaborative way. If the parent says "Yes," perhaps a discussion of obstacles that interfered with the parent's ability to do the Daily Behavioral Chart would be useful. Obstacles could range from a parent "forgetting" to "not having enough time" to "feeling too depressed lately." The practitioner and parent could then brainstorm strategies to deal with these obstacles (see Chapter 9 for more ideas on overcoming obstacles).

Preparation for change should be thought of a as a fluid, somewhat elusive part of an intervention. **A practitioner may need to alternate between skills training and preparation for change over the course of working with a family.**

TRAINING METHODS

This book describes many different skills training procedures (Success Plans) that can be used by parents. The practitioner can help the parents learn these skills through behavioral training techniques. Behavioral techniques include all or some of the following methods:

1. **Socratic questioning.** Do not tell the parents and/or child what to do. Instead, guide them using Socratic questioning to "discover" areas of focus the parents and/or child think are important.
2. **Didactic explanation.** Fully explain the skill within a Success Plan.
3. **Modeling/demonstration.** Act out the skill and allow the parents and/or child to observe.
4. **Role playing.** Instruct the parents and/or child to act out and demonstrate how they might implement the skill.
5. **Apply skills in the session.** Look for opportunities to prompt the parents and/or child to use the skills in session with real problems that come up while meeting.
6. **Have parents and/or child "teach" each other.** One of the best ways to learn is to teach. Ask the parents and/or child to teach each other about a specific skill they have learned.
7. **Application in real-life environment.** Instruct the parents and/or child to use the new skill in real life.
8. **Homework.** Give the parents and/or child specific homework assignments utilizing the corresponding form or chart that goes with a particular skill.
9. **Periodic review.** Over the course of intervention, review and evaluate the progress of the parents and/or child.

The practitioner can use many of these training methods to help parents and family members learn skills.

The practitioner will also have to determine whether to deliver skills training to parents via family or group sessions. Family sessions have the advantage of being able to tailor the content of what is presented to the unique needs of the family. Family sessions might be a better match for some parents who would not like the social nature of a group or who cannot accommodate the scheduled time of a group or find transportation to the session. Parent groups are economical for the practitioner who needs to serve many families. Some parents also enjoy the support they derive from discussing "war stories" of raising children with other parents, and they can give each other emotional support better than a practitioner because they've "been there." It is a judgment call that practitioners need to make as to what mode of service delivery to make use of based on the unique features of their employment and the families they are serving. Either mode of delivery will work if the above behavioral training techniques are employed.

PROCEDURES FOR CONDUCTING FAMILY SESSIONS

The first consideration is **who should be invited?** Obviously, the parents and the child should be there, and there may be advantages to having siblings or extended family members attend. Generally speaking, siblings who are affected by or affect the child in a significant manner and are over the age of about 5 or 6 years can benefit to varying degrees from the family sessions. The sibling could learn similar skills, and the parents could guide the child and the sibling together in their application. There may be situations also in which a child spends a lot of time with extended family members (e.g., grandparents). It may be helpful to involve extended family members in the training sessions so that they can better understand the child and be able to guide the child in skills development.

One way to deliver skills training with families is to train parents to train the child. The goal with this delivery method is to enable the parents to train and facilitate the child in skills development. The practitioner would first meet with the parents to instruct, model, role play, plan, and so forth. Once the practitioner has trained the parents, the child would be invited into the session. Then the parents would instruct, model, role play, plan, and so forth with the child to train him in the skill.

Another way to deliver skills training with families is first to train the child in child-focused skills and then train parents to prompt and reinforce the child at home. The goal of this delivery method is to help the parents learn how to facilitate skills development at home after the practitioner has trained the child. The practitioner would first meet with the child to instruct, model, role play, and plan regarding a certain skills training area. In this instance the practitioner would use the instructions from the Skills Training book as a basis for training the child. For example, if the practitioner is training the child in anger management skills, the Anger Management Success Plan instructions in Chapter 3 could be used by the practitioner. After the child has been trained, the parents would be invited into the session. If the child is able, ask him to give an explanation of the skills training procedures to the parent. The practitioner would also instruct, model, role play, and plan with the parents as to how they can guide the child in using the skill at home.

A final way to deliver skills training with families is to work with all family members simultaneously. The goal of this delivery method is to train family members together in skills development and to train the parents to facilitate skills deployment at home. This method may be preferred when the focus is on family interaction skills (e.g., Chapter 8) and/or when working with an older child/teen. The practitioner would meet with the family members to instruct, model, role play, and plan regarding a certain skill and how parents can facilitate skill use at home.

In most instances, it is recommended that the practitioner initially **contract with the family for about six to ten sessions.** Usually, it's best to conduct the first four to six sessions once a week and then spread out the remaining sessions over an extended period of time to give the families enough time to practice the skills. Even after the six to ten sessions, it is common to continue to monitor the child and family's progress for an extended period of time. Follow-up sessions can be offered in accordance with the progress being made and maintained by the child and family.

PROCEDURES FOR CONDUCTING PARENT GROUP SESSIONS

Make sure preparation for change has been completed with all parents individually before enrolling them in parent groups. This is important so that all parents in attendance are ready to learn and develop skills. If one parent or couple is not ready, it could result in their dropping out, or, if they regularly attend, it could have a negative effect on the other participating group members who are farther along in the change process.

The **number of participants and practitioners** for a group depends on the setting and the goals of the practitioner. The ideal is to limit the size of the group to the parents of about six to eight children. Two practitioners are best to conduct this type of group, but one practitioner could work with a group of parents if staffing resources are limited. In a larger setting (e.g., school, community center), large numbers of parents could receive training. In this context, the training would have more of a large group "workshop" format, but allow time at the end for small break-out group discussions. One practitioner could conduct the large group presentation, but there would need to be additional practitioners in each small break-out group.

The **methods the practitioner uses in conducting the parent group sessions** are important to consider. A good time sequence is to allocate about 15 minutes for introduction/check-in, about 30–45 minutes for didactic instruction/modeling/role playing, and about 30–45 minutes for parents to discuss and practice the skills presented in that session. The notion of providing parental emotional support cannot be overemphasized. Although most of the training is focused on skill acquisition, be sure to leave enough time for the parents to discuss their own individual concerns and problems. Many parents comment that the emotional support they receive as part of the group experience is very important and helpful to them. Some parents are intimidated or uncomfortable with role playing in front of others. It is a good idea to make it clear that role playing is optional and that no one has to do anything that is uncomfortable for him or her. Try to make the group experience as enjoyable and interesting as possible.

The exact number of parent group sessions may vary depending on the goals of the practitioners and the nature of the parents in the group. The number of sessions can therefore vary according to what the leader elects to cover. The author's experience suggests that **about 10 parent group sessions are sufficient and practical to cover a well-planned group program.** It's always a good idea to allow occasional sessions to review previously learned material. Follow-up with families can occur in family sessions once the parent group is over.

One drawback to the parent group training format is that it is hard to individualize the area of focus and corresponding Success Plans to each family participating in the group. A "cafeteria" procedure works best and involves presenting an overview of selected Success Plans from the book and then helping individual families within the group choose the specific Success Plan(s) that fits them best.

SENSITIVITY TO MULTICULTURAL ISSUES

Efforts should be made to make interventions compatible with families of varying cultural backgrounds. Individuals from diverse cultural groups might differ in terms of language, structure of the family and community, views on child development and parenting, and help-seeking behavior. A practitioner should take cultural considerations into account and adjust delivery of skills training accordingly. It is beyond the scope of this chapter to review all concepts and procedures involved in delivery of multiculturally sensitive services. Interested readers are referred to Boyd-Franklin (2003) and Dumas, Rollock, Prinz, Hops, and Blechman (1999) for more on this topic. Several suggestions are offered, however, based on the author's knowledge and experience in delivering skills training to children and families of different cultural backgrounds.

One procedure that helps to promote multicultural sensitivity is to **emphasize collaboration.** This involves actively listening to each family, presenting multiple intervention options, and seeking as much input from family members as possible. This will insure use of skills training procedures that are meaningful and respectful of participating families.

Framing the skills training intervention in developmental terms may also assist families from varied cultural groups in acceptance of the intervention. The basic idea is to describe skills training as a method to help children enhance their level of development. Although there are culturally influenced differences in how children develop, there are also many "universal" stages of child development that seem to cut across cultures. For example, most children learn basic social skills in their preschool years, although there may be subtle differences in exactly what social skills are learned for a particular cultural group. Parents should be taught basic skills and encouraged to **make modifications as needed to fit their beliefs, values, and goals as shaped by their cultural background.**

The author attempted to make the text of Skills Training book sensitive to cultural issues. Many of the illustrations are either "acultural" (e.g., circle faces) or depict individuals of different cultural backgrounds. The text also has before-and-after vignettes that are intended to apply to people from different cultures.

PROCEDURES FOR USING THIS BOOK IN SKILLS TRAINING INTERVENTIONS

This book can be used in a number of different ways depending on a particular family's needs and the goals for the intervention. The practitioner could provide the entire book or the opportunity to purchase the book to a family. **Parents could be asked to read chapters before and/or after a session to aid in the training process.** Alternatively, because the author and publisher grant permission to reproduce any chart from Chapters 3–8 for skills training purposes, the practitioner could **provide copies of selected charts to a family.**

This book is written in a fairly sophisticated manner that may be difficult for some parents. The author elected to write in a thorough and somewhat detailed manner to enhance parents' understanding and execution of the skills on their own. Unfortunately, not all parents can benefit from this due to limited reading ability. **In cases where parents have limited reading ability, the practitioner could emphasize verbal instructions and modeling as a way of explaining procedures.** The practitioner could still use the charts from the book with these parents. The charts are, for the most part, fairly easy to comprehend and could be used with less educated parents. In particular, the visually oriented charts may be of greatest utility for these families.

FOLLOW-UP WITH FAMILIES

It is not uncommon when using a skills training approach to follow families for months, or even years, by conducting periodic booster sessions now and then. This follow-up is a critical component in working with families. The practitioner should assume that development of skills takes a long time and that there is significant risk of relapse. **By having these periodic reviews and follow-up sessions, the practitioner can monitor the family's progress, refocus the family if necessary, and/or review previously learned skills.** Extended follow-up can be accomplished by intermittently meeting with the family (e.g., several sessions per year, once a month) or by asking the family to contact the practitioner should future problems arise.

Ideas for Rewarding Child Behavior

Throughout this book, various skills training exercises or charts make reference to rewarding a child to motivate learning and use of new skills. This Appendix presents specific ideas on how to select and use rewards for children in skills training.

The first step in selecting a reward is to **ask your child what is rewarding to him.** The Reward Ideas chart (at the end of the Appendix) is a good place to start. It may be helpful to review this chart with your child and select a reward. In any event, you and he should discuss the reward. Make sure it will really motivate him and catch his interest. Next, and equally as important, **make sure the reward is realistic for you to give.**

It is important to vary the reward to keep a child's interest. A child can become used to, and bored by, the same old reward. A powerful way to vary the reward is to use a reward menu. This involves creating a variety of rewards (10–15 rewards are preferable) and writing them down on a menu. A "mystery reward," where the child earns something without knowing what it is, is also very motivating for most children. When your child meets his behavior expectation, he would then be able to select one reward from the reward menu. If a child wants to earn a big reward, such as a CD player or going to a concert, you could use a token system. Each day he could earn tokens to be exchanged later for a bigger reward. See the example Reward Menus for more ideas (at the end of the Appendix).

Rewards don't always have to be "extras." It's OK to take away privileges your child may take for granted and then allow him to "earn them back." For example, a child may find a video game rewarding. A parent could take this privilege away and make the child adhere to a behavior expectation to earn video game time. Earning a privilege that may be taken for granted can be rewarding to a child.

Try to emphasize social and privilege rewards over material rewards. Material rewards (e.g., toys, cars, money) often lose their reinforcing value and are very expensive. As was mentioned earlier, many children benefit from more involvement with their parents. Rewards involving time and activities with caregivers can be reinforcing and promote involvement at the same time.

After the reward is selected, make sure the child knows what he has to do to earn it. Many of the procedures discussed in Chapters 3–6 state explicitly what a child must do to earn rewards. The link between the child's behavior and the reward needs to be clear to the child.

REWARD IDEAS

1. Favorite dessert

2. Favorite meal

3. Special snack

4. Small toy

5. Sports equipment

6. CDs/tapes

7. Rent special DVDs

8. Furnishing for room

9. Attention

10. Praise

11. Display work on refrigerator

12. Special privileges

13. Private time in room

14. Special TV, computer, or video game privileges

15. Stay up late

16. Have a friend over for dinner or overnight

17. Special time with one parent

18. Go to a movie

19. Go to a concert

20. Go on a special trip

21. Attend a sporting event

22. Camping

23. Traveling

24. Have a party

25. Tokens for general exchange

Note: Make sure the reward is motivating for the child and is realistic for the parent to give the child.

EXAMPLE: REWARD MENUS

For an 8-year-old

_____   Use of TV for 2 hours during 1 day

_____   Use of computer video game for 2 hours during 1 day

_____   Take a 30-minute walk with Mom

_____   Play one-on-one basketball with Dad for 30 minutes

_____   Special snack at bedtime

_____   Dad cooks a favorite meal

_____   Get to have a friend over for supper

_____   Earn 1 token per day (exchange 5 tokens for a movie or 7 tokens for 1 day fishing outing with parent)

_____   Mystery reward

For a 16-year-old (some of above might work)

_____   Extra driving privileges for a day

_____   Stay out 30 minutes late

_____   Get to stay on phone extra 30 minutes past phone curfew

_____   Earn 1 token per day (exchange 5 tokens for a concert)

From _Skills Training for Children with Behavior Problems: A Parent and Practitioner Guidebook_ (revised edition) by Michael L. Bloomquist. Copyright 2006 by The Guilford Press. Permission to photocopy this chart is granted to purchasers of this book for personal or professional use only (see copyright page for details).

Suggested Readings

American Psychiatric Association. (2000). *Diagnostic and statistical manual of mental disorders* (4th ed., text rev.). Washington, DC: Author.

Anastopoulos, A. D., Shelton, T. L., DuPaul, G. J., & Guevremont, D. C. (1993). Parent training for ADHD: Its impact on parent functioning. *Journal of Abnormal Child Psychology, 21*, 581–596.

Assemany, A. E., & McIntosh, D. E. (2002). Negative treatment outcomes of behavioral parent training programs. *Psychology in the Schools, 39*, 209–219.

Barkley, R. A. (1997). *Defiant children: A clinician's manual for assessment and parent training* (2nd ed.). New York: Guilford Press.

Barkley, R. A. (2000). *Taking charge of ADHD: The complete, authoritative guide for parents* (rev ed.). New York: Guilford Press.

Barkley, R. A. (2006). *Attention-defici;t hyperactivity disorder: A handbook for diagnosis and treatment* (3rd ed.). New York: Guilford Press.

Barkley, R. A., & Benton, C. M. (1998). *Your defiant child*. New York: Guilford Press.

Barkley, R. A., Edwards, G., Laneri, M., Fletcher, K., & Metevia, L. (2001). The efficacy of problem-solving communication training alone, behavior management training alone, and their combination for parent–adolescent conflict in teenagers with ADHD and ODD. *Journal of Consulting and Clinical Psychology, 69*, 926–941.

Barkley, R. A., Edwards, G. H., & Robin, A. L. (1999). *Defiant teens: A clinician's manual for assessment and family intervention*. New York: Guilford Press.

Beelmann, A., Pfingsten, U., & Losel, F. (1994). Effects of training social competence in children: A meta-analysis of recent evaluation studies. *Journal of Clinical Child Psychology, 23*, 260–271.

Bierman, K. L., Greenberg, M. T., & Conduct Problems Prevention Research Group. (1996). Social skills training in the Fast Track program. In R. D. Peters & R. J. McMahon (Eds.), *Preventing childhood disorders, substance abuse, and delinquency* (pp. 65–89). Thousand Oaks, CA: Sage.

Bloomquist, M. L. (1996). *Skills training for children with behavior disorders: A parent and therapist guidebook.* New York: Guilford Press.

Bloomquist, M. L., & Schnell, S. V. (2002). *Helping children with aggression and conduct problems: Best practices for intervention.* New York: Guilford Press.

Boyd-Franklin, N. (2003). *Black families in therapy* (2nd ed.). New York: Guilford Press.

Braswell, L., & Bloomquist, M. L. (1991). *Cognitive-behavioral therapy with ADHD children: Child, family, and school interventions.* New York: Guilford Press.

Brestan, E. V., & Eyberg, S. M. (1998). Effective psychosocial treatments of conduct-disordered children and adolescents: 29 years, 82 studies, and 5272 kids. *Journal of Clinical Child Psychology, 27,* 180–189.

Brinkmeyer, M. Y., & Eyberg, S. M. (2003). Parent–child interaction therapy for oppositional children. In A. E. Kazdin & J. R. Weisz (Eds.), *Evidence-based psychotherapies for children and adolescents* (pp. 204–223). New York: Guilford Press.

Cavell, T. A. (2000). *Working with parents of aggressive children: A practitioner's guide.* Washington, DC: American Psychological Association.

Cummings, E. M., Davies, P. T., & Campbell, S. B. (2000). *Developmental psychopathology and family process: Theory, research, and clinical implications.* New York: Guilford Press.

Dishon, T. J., & Kavanagh, K. (2003). *Intervening in adolescent problem behavior: A family-centered approach.* New York: Guilford Press.

Dumas, J. E., Rollock, D., Prinz, R. J., Hops, H., & Blechman, E. A. (1999). Cultural sensitivity: Problems and solutions in applied and preventive intervention. *Applied and Preventive Psychology, 8,* 175–196.

Eyberg, S. M., & Boggs, S. R. (1998). Parent–child interaction therapy: A psychosocial intervention for treatment of young conduct-disordered children. In J. M. Briesmeister & C. E. Schaefer (Eds.), *Handbook of parent training: Parents as co-therapists for children's behavior problems* (2nd ed., pp. 61–97). New York: Wiley.

Eyberg, S. M., Boggs, S. R., & Algina, J. (1995). Parent–child interaction therapy: A psychosocial model for the treatment of young children with conduct problem behavior and their families. *Psychopharmacology Bulletin, 31,* 83–91.

Faraone, S. V. (2003). *Straight talk about your child's mental health: What to do when something seems wrong.* New York: Guilford Press.

Fiese, B. H., Tomcho, T. J., Douglas, M., Josephs, K., Poltrock, S., & Baker, T. (2002). A review of 50 years of research on naturally occurring family routines and rituals: Cause for celebration? *Journal of Family Psychology, 16,* 381–390.

Forgatch, M., & Patterson, G. R. (1989). *Parents and adolescents living together: Part 2. Family problem solving.* Eugene, OR: Castalia.

Frey, K. S., Hirschstein, M. K., & Guzzo, B. A. (2000). Second step: Preventing aggression by promoting social competence. *Journal of Emotional and Behavioral Disorders, 8,* 102–112.

Greenberg, M. T., Kusche, C. A., Cook, E. T., & Quamma, J. P. (1995). Promoting emotional competence in school-aged children: The effects of the PATHS curriculum. *Development and Psychopathology, 7,* 117–136.

Greene, R. W. (1998). *The explosive child.* New York: HarperCollins.

Greene, R. W., Ablon, J. S., Monteaux, M. C., Goring, J. C., Henin, A., & Raezer, L. (2004). Effectiveness of collaborative problem-solving in affectively dysregulated children with Oppositional Defiant Disorder: Initial findings. *Journal of Consulting and Clinical Psychology, 72,* 1157–1164.

Grossman, D. C., Neckerman, H. J., Koepsell, T. D., Liu, P. -Y., Asher, K. N., Beland, K., Frey, K., & Rivara, F. P. (1997). Effectiveness of a violence prevention curriculum among children in elementary school: A randomized controlled trial. *Journal of the American Medical Association, 277,* 1605–1611.

Henggeler, S. W., & Lee, T. (2003). Multisystemic treatment of serious clinical problems. In A. E. Kazdin & J. R. Weisz (Eds.), *Evidence-based psychotherapies for children and adolescents* (pp. 301–324). New York: Guilford Press.

Henggeler, S. W., Schoenwald, S. K., Borduin, C. M., Rowland, M. D., & Cunningham, P. B. (1998). *Multisystemic treatment of antisocial behavior in children and adolescents.* New York: Guilford Press.

Hinshaw, S. P. (2000). Attention-deficit/hyperactivity disorder: The search for viable treatments. In P. C. Kendall (Ed.), *Child and adolescent therapy* (2nd ed., pp. 88–128). New York: Guilford Press.

Hinshaw, S. P., Henker, B., & Whalen, C. K. (1984a). Cognitive-behavioral and pharmacologic interventions for hyperactive boys: Comparative and combined effects. *Journal of Consulting and Clinical Psychology, 52,* 739–749.

Hinshaw, S. P., Henker, B., & Whalen, C. K. (1984b). Self-control in hyperactive boys in anger-inducing situations: Effects of cognitive-behavioral training and of methylphenidate. *Journal of Abnormal Child Psychology, 12,* 55–77.

Hudley, C. A., Britsch, B., Wakefield, W. D., Smith, T., Demorat, M., & Cho, S. (1998). An attribution retraining program to reduce aggression in elementary school students. *Psychology in the Schools, 35,* 271–282.

Hudley, C. A., & Graham, S. (1993). An attributional intervention to reduce peer-directed aggression among African-American boys. *Child Development, 64,* 124–138.

Kam, C., Greenberg, M. T., & Kusche, C. A. (2003). Sustained effects of the PATHS curriculum on the social and psychological adjustment of children in special education. *Journal of Emotional and Behavioral Disorders, 12,* 66–78.

Kazdin, A. E. (1996a). Dropping out of child psychotherapy: Issues for research and implications for practice. *Clinical Child Psychology and Psychiatry, 1,* 133–156.

Kazdin, A. E. (1996b). Problem solving and parent management in treating aggressive and antisocial children. In E. S. Hibbs & P. S. Jensen (Eds.), *Psychosocial treatments for child and adolescent disorders* (pp. 377–408). Washington, DC: American Psychological Association.

Kazdin, A. E. (1997). Practitioner review: Psychosocial treatments for conduct disorder in children. *Journal of Child Psychology and Psychiatry, 38,* 161–178.

Kazdin, A. E. (2003). Problem-solving skills training and parent management training for conduct disorder. In A. E. Kazdin & J. R. Weisz (Eds.), *Evidence-based psychotherapies for children and adolescents* (pp. 241–262). New York: Guilford Press.

Kendall, P. C., & Braswell, L. (1993). *Cognitive-behavioral therapy for impulsive children* (2nd ed.). New York: Guilford Press.

Larson, J., & Lochman, J. E. (2002). *Helping school children cope with anger: A cognitive-behavioral intervention.* New York: Guilford Press.

Lochman, J. E., Barry, T. D., & Pardini, D. A. (2003). Anger control training for aggressive youth. In A. E. Kazdin & J. R. Weisz (Eds.), *Evidence-based psychotherapies for children and adolescents* (pp. 263–281). New York: Guilford Press.

Masten, A. S., & Coatsworth, J. D. (1998). The development of competence in favorable and unfavorable environments: Lessons from research on successful children. *American Psychologist, 53,* 205–220.

McFadyen-Ketchum, S. A., & Dodge, K. A. (1998). Problems in social relationships. In E. J. Mash & R. A. Barkley (Eds.), *Treatment of childhood disorders* (2nd ed., pp. 338–365). New York: Guilford Press.

McGoldrick, M., Giordano, J., & Garcia-Preto, N. (2005). Overview: Ethnicity and family therapy. In M. McGoldrick, J. Giordano, & N. Garcia-Preto (Eds.), *Ethnicity and family therapy* (3rd ed., pp. 1–40). New York: Guilford Press.

McMahon, R. J., & Forehand, R. L. (2003). *Helping the noncompliant child: Family-based treatment for oppositional behavior* (2nd ed.). New York: Guilford Press.

McMahon, R. J., Slough, N. M., & Conduct Problems Prevention. Research Group. (1996). Family-based intervention in the Fast Track program. In R. D. Peters & R. J. McMahon (Eds.), *Preventing childhood disorders, substance abuse, and delinquency* (pp. 90–110). Thousand Oaks, CA: Sage.

Morrissey-Kane, E., & Prinz, R. J. (1999). Engagement in child and adolescent treatment: The role of parental cognitions and attributions. *Clinical Child and Family Psychology Review, 2,* 183–198.

Patterson, G. R. (1975). *Families: Applications of social learning to family life* (rev. ed.). Champaign, IL: Research Press.

Patterson, G. R. (1976). *Living with children: New methods for parents and teachers* (rev. ed.). Champaign, IL: Research Press.

Patterson, G. R., Cobb, J. A., & Ray, R. S. (1973). A social engineering technology for retraining the families of aggressive boys. In H. E. Adams & I. P. Unikel (Eds.), *Issues and trends in behavior therapy* (pp. 139–210). Springfield, IL: Charles C Thomas.

Patterson, G. R., & Forgatch, M. (1987). *Parents and adolescents living together: Part 1. The basics.* Eugene, OR: Castalia.

Patterson, G. R., & Gullion, M. E. (1968). *Living with children: New methods for parents and teachers.* Champaign, IL: Research Press.

Patterson, G. R., Reid, J. B., Jones, R. R., & Conger R. E. (1975). *A social learning approach to family intervention: Vol. 1. Families with aggressive children.* Eugene, OR: Castalia.

Pelham, W. E., Wheeler, T., & Chronis, A. (1998). Empirically supported psychosocial treatments for attention deficit hyperactivity disorder. *Journal of Clinical Child Psychology, 27,* 190–205.

Prinz, R. J., Blechman, E. A., & Dumas, J. E. (1994). An evaluation of peer-coping skills training for childhood aggression. *Journal of Clinical Child Psychology, 23,* 193–203.

Prinz, R. J., & Miller, G. E. (1996). Parental engagement in interventions for children at risk for Conduct Disorder. In R. D. Peters & R. J. McMahon (Eds.), *Preventing childhood disorders, substance abuse, and delinquency* (pp. 161–183). Thousand Oaks, CA: Sage.

Quinn, M. M., Kavale, K. A., Mathur, S. R., Rutherford, R. B., & Forness, S. R. (1999). A meta-analysis of social skill interventions for students with emotional or behavioral disorders. *Journal of Emotional and Behavioral Disorders, 7,* 54–64.

Rathvon, N. (1999). *Effective school interventions.* New York: Guilford Press.

Robin, A. L., & Foster, S. L. (1989). *Negotiating parent–adolescent conflict: A behavioral–family systems approach.* New York: Guilford Press.

Roth, A., & Fonagy, P. (2005). *What works for whom?: A critical review of psychotherapy research* (2nd ed.). New York: Guilford Press.

Sanders, M. R. (1999). Triple P—Positive Parenting Program: Towards an empirically validated multilevel parenting and family support strategy for prevention of behavior and emotional problems in children. *Clinical Child and Family Psychology Review, 2,* 71–90.

Serketich, W. J., & Dumas, J. E. (1996). The effectiveness of behavioral parent training to modify antisocial behavior in children: A meta-analysis. *Behavior Therapy, 27,* 171–186.

Stark, K. D., Boswell Sander, J., Yancy, M. G., Bronik, M. D., & Hoke, J. A. (2000). Treatment of depression in childhood and adolescence: Cognitive-behavioral procedures for the individual and family. In P. C. Kendall (Ed.), *Child and adolescent therapy: Cognitive-behavioral procedures* (2nd ed., pp. 173–234). New York: Guilford Press.

Taylor, T. K., Eddy, J. M., & Biglan, A. (1999). Interpersonal skills training to reduce aggressive and delinquent behavior: Limited evidence and the need for an evidence-based system of care. *Clinical Child and Family Psychology Review, 2,* 169–182.

Tynan, W. D., Schuman, W., & Lampert, N. (1999). Concurrent parent and child therapy groups for externalizing disorders: From the laboratory to the world of managed care. *Cognitive and Behavioral Practice, 6,* 3–9.

Walker, H. M., Colvin, G., & Ramsey, E. (1995). *Antisocial behavior in school: Strategies and best practices.* Pacific Grove, CA: Brooks/Cole.

Webster-Stratton, C. (1992). *The incredible years: A troubleshooting guide for parents and children ages 3–8*. Toronto: Umbrella Press.

Webster-Stratton, C. (1996). Early intervention with videotape modeling: Programs for families of children with oppositional defiant or conduct disorder. In E. S. Hibbs & P. S. Jensen (Eds.), *Psychosocial treatments for child and adolescent disorders* (pp. 435–474). Washington, DC: American Psychological Association.

Webster-Stratton, C., & Reid, M. J. (2003). The Incredible Years parents, teachers, and child training series: A multifaceted treatment approach for young children with conduct problems. In A. E. Kazdin & J. R. Weisz (Eds.), *Evidence-based psychotherapies for children and adolescents* (pp. 224–240). New York: Guilford Press.

Weisz, J. R., Weiss, B., Han, S. S., Granger, D. A., & Morton, T. (1995). Effects of psychotherapy with children and adolescents revisited: A meta-analysis of treatment outcome studies. *Psychological Bulletin, 117*, 450–468.

Index